Promoting Health and Equity: From Policy to Action
Cases from the Western Pacific Region

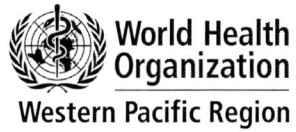

March 2009

Photo credits: Steven Nowakowski (2006) p. viii, Andrea Fisch (1988) p. 46, Elson T. Elizaga (2006) p. 128, John McCombe (undated) p. 98

WHO Library Cataloguing in Publication Data

Promoting Health and Equity : From Policy to Action : Cases from the Western Pacific Region

1. Health services accessibility. 2. Health policy. 3. Evidence-based practice. 4. Western Pacific

ISBN 987 92 9061 427 2   (NLM Classification: W 76)

© World Health Organization 2009
All rights reserved.

The designations employed and the presentation of the material in this publication do not imply the expression of any opinion whatsoever on the part of the World Health Organization concerning the legal status of any country, territory, city or area or of its authorities, or concerning the delimitation of its frontiers or boundaries. Dotted lines on maps represent approximate border lines for which there may not yet be full agreement.

The mention of specific companies or of certain manufacturers' products does not imply that they are endorsed or recommended by the World Health Organization in preference to others of a similar nature that are not mentioned. Errors and omissions excepted, the names of proprietary products are distinguished by initial capital letters.

The World Health Organization does not warrant that the information contained in this publication is complete and correct and shall not be liable for any damages incurred as a result of its use.

Publications of the World Health Organization can be obtained from WHO Press, World Health Organization, 20 Avenue Appia, 1211 Geneva 27, Switzerland (tel: +41 22 791 2476; fax: +41 22 791 4857; e-mail: bookorders@who.int). Requests for permission to reproduce WHO publications, in part or in whole, or to translate them – whether for sale or for noncommercial distribution – should be addressed to WHO Press, at the above address (fax: +41 22 791 4806; e-mail: permissions@who.int). For WHO Western Pacific Regional Publications, request for permission to reproduce should be addressed to Publications Office, World Health Organization, Regional Office for the Western Pacific, P.O. Box 2932, 1000, Manila, Philippines, fax: +632 521 1036, e-mail: publications@wpro.who.int

Table of Contents

Acronyms	vi
Improving health equity through the use of evidence: cases from the Western Pacific Region	1
Health financing strategies to improve access to health services for the poor in Cambodia: from pilot to policy and action— A case study of Health Equity Funds	29
Research, intervention design and policy implementation of the New Rural Cooperative Medical Scheme in Shandong, China	47
Health Care Fund for the Poor in Viet Nam: how evidence and politics came together	63
Scaling up primary health care in the Lao People's Democratic Republic using evidence from a long-term primary health care development project	81
Promoting health equity: evidence, policy and action— The New Zealand experience	99
The development and targeting of malaria control interventions for populations in high transmission areas of Cambodia: the influence of research on policy and practice	115
Public-private mix DOTS: a strategy to engage all health care providers in tuberculosis control and significantly increase access to DOTS services in the Philippines	129
Geographic equity in distribution of scarce dialysis resources in Malaysia	143
Promoting health equity through capacity building of primary health care workers in Mongolia	157

Acronyms

ADB	Asian Development Bank
AIDS	Acquired immunodeficiency syndrome
AusAID	Australian Agency for International Development
CBHI	Community-based health insurance
CDC	Centers for Disease Control
CHS	Commune health station
CMBS	Cambodia Malaria Baseline Survey
CNM	National Malaria Centre
CUP	Comprehensive and Unified Policy for Tuberculosis Control
DfID	Department for International Development
DOT	Directly-observed treatment
DOTS	Directly-observed treatment, short-course therapy
DPMU	District project management unit
DRF	Drug revolving fund
EC	European Commission
EDAT	Early diagnosis and appropriate treatment
EPI	Expanded programme on immunization
EVIPNet	Evidence-Informed Policy Network
GDP	Gross domestic product
GIS	Geographic information system
GRET	Groupe de Recherche et d'Echanges Technologiques
HEF	Health equity fund
HEPR	Hunger Eradication and Poverty Reduction programme
HIS	Health information system
HNZ	Housing New Zealand
HSPI	Health Strategy and Policy Institute
HSRP	Health Sector Reform Project
HSSP	National Health Strategic Plan 2003-2007
ITN	Insecticide-treated bednet
JICA	Japan International Cooperation Agency
LLIN	Long-lasting insecticidal net
MAF	Medical assistance fund
MDG	Millennium Development Goal
MSF	Médecins Sans Frontières
NCMS	New Cooperative Medical Service
NGO	Non-governmental organization
NGPES	National Growth and Poverty Eradication Strategy
NHC	National Health Committee

NHSS	National Health Service Survey
NPRS	National Poverty Reduction Strategy 2003-2005
pACT	Pre-packaged artemisinin-based combination therapy
PHC	Primary health care
PhilCAT	Philippine Coalition against Tuberculosis
PhilHealth	Philippine Health Insurance Corporation
PhilTIPS	Philippine Tuberculosis Initiative for the Private Sector
PHO	Primary Health Organisation
PMU	Project management unit
PPMD	Public-Private Mix DOTS
PPMU	Provincial project management unit
PPP	Purchasing power parity
PRSP	Poverty Reduction Strategy Paper
RDT	Rapid diagnostic test
RII	Relative index of inequality
RM	Malaysian ringgit
SARS	Severe acute respiratory syndrome
SCA	Save the Children Australia
SEDP6	6th Socio-economic Development Plan
SII	Slope index of inequality
SRD	Standardized rate difference
SRR	Standardized rate ratio
SWAp	Sector-wide approach
TB	Tuberculosis
TBA	Traditional birth attendant
TFR	Total fertility rate
TWG-H	Technical Working Group-Health
UNICEF	United Nations Children's Fund
VHLSS	Vietnam Household Living Standard Survey
VHV	Village health volunteer
VND	Vietnamese Dong
VSS	Vietnam Social Security
WHO	World Health Organization

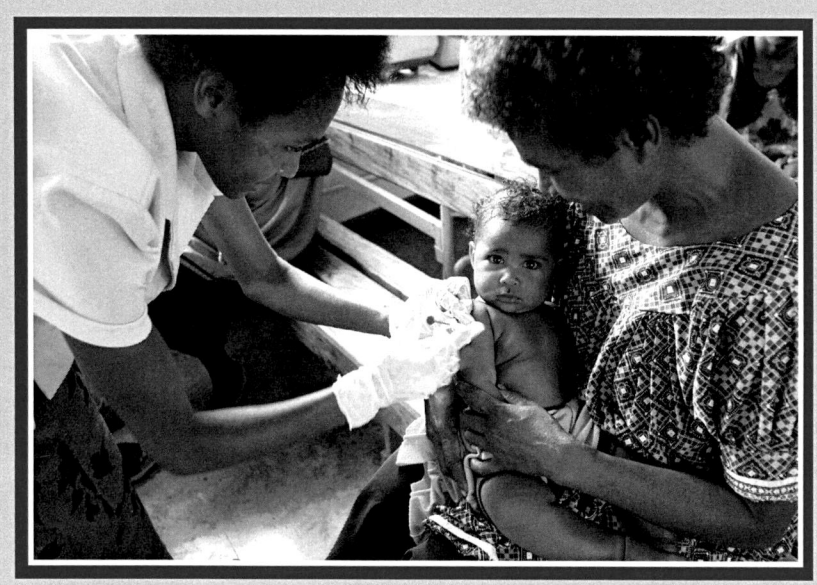

Improving health equity through the use of evidence: cases from the Western Pacific Region

Steve Fabricant[1]

Introduction

Health equity and the barriers to achieving it in developing countries have been a major subject of research for many years, resulting in a growing evidence base on policies and actions to promote health equity. Despite efforts over the past two decades, the evidence shows that inequalities are increasing rather than decreasing in many countries. This may partly be due to faulty policy decisions that have increased some of the barriers to access to health services faced by the poor. It has become clear that a better evidence-based approach to health policy is needed, with equity as its focus.

At the same time, understanding is also inadequate on how the growing evidence base on promoting equity in health can be best used by policy-makers. Health policy development in countries is increasingly supported by research, involving a range of stakeholders including academic institutions, government think tanks, NGOs and consumer groups. Partners from other international organizations, academia, and research networks are also engaged in strengthening the evidence base for health policy and action, including that focusing on equity-, gender-, and poverty-related issues in health. However, the links between evidence and policy-making are inconsistent and variable. There is, thus, still a need for stronger links between evidence and health policy-making and implementation.

The World Health Organization (WHO) is increasingly asked to help strengthen mechanisms that link research and policy-making in developing countries. For example, in May 2005, resolution WHA 58.34 called for better use of health research and health information, as well as better knowledge management, to support evidence-informed health policy and practice, specifically requesting WHO to assist in the development of more effective mechanisms to bridge the divide between knowledge generation and its use, including the translation of health research findings into policy and practice. At the fifty-seventh session of the WHO Regional Committee held in September 2006, a ministerial round table discussion was held on the topic Translation of Research into Policy and Health Care Practice, and WHO was requested to lead efforts to strengthen the capacity for better utilization of research results in national health policy-making. This is one of the strategic directions for WHO in the period 2008–2013.

---

[1] Consultant, World Health Organization Western Pacific Regional Office

To respond in part to this need, the WHO Western Pacific Regional Office convened the High-Level Meeting on Promoting Health Equity: Evidence, Policy and Action, from 16 to 18 October 2007 in Phnom Penh, hosted by the Royal Government of Cambodia, with the objective of giving participants the opportunity to exchange experiences in evidence-based policy-making, and to identify ways to promote the more systematic use of equity research in health policy and action.

Health ministries and other stakeholders engaged in the evidence-to-policy process in the Western Pacific Region were invited to submit case studies that illustrate how the process has worked in their country. Nine cases were presented, representing experiences in eight countries. In the discussions that followed, participants identified key factors that can strengthen the capacity for evidence-based policy-making and develop a culture of investing in and acting upon information and evidence. The meeting also provided useful ideas for promoting evidence-based debate, analysis and policy development for health equity over the longer term.

This book compiles all nine cases. This introductory chapter comprises a synthesis of the cases and the lessons learned from them. Comparing and contrasting the different cases, it identifies key factors that stimulate policy-relevant research and better use of evidence for policy-making. These lessons can be especially valuable for developing countries, where resources are limited and better understanding of the trade-offs implied by alternative policy choices is needed.

Equity and barriers to access to health services

Overall gains in health can occur amid persistent, and even widening, inequalities between socio-economic groups and areas. To narrow health gaps under a condition of resource constraints requires improving the health of the poorest and doing so at a rate that outstrips that of the wider population. Effective pro-equity health policy can achieve absolute and relative improvement in the health of the poorest groups, and in the factors that determine their access to health care and their exposure to risk factors.

It is now well understood that poor, vulnerable and socially excluded groups have a higher burden of disease, while at the same time having worse access to and lower utilization of health services, a phenomenon described by the "inverse care law".[1] Evidence from the Western Pacific region presented at the High-Level Meeting confirmed that households in the lowest income quintile, and those in rural areas, use fewer health services than those in higher income quintiles or in urban areas. These groups face financial, geographical, and socio-cultural barriers to equitable access to health services. Health systems can attempt to reduce these obstacles, but often fail to respond adequately.

The tools policy-makers have at their disposal for reducing these access barriers include directing public subsidies to poor and excluded groups, either spatially or by targeting specific health conditions, making greater use of existing private sector providers, and monitoring health system performance. However, public subsidies have been shown to actually benefit the better-off more than the poor, unless there is an explicit pro-poor focus, accompanied by effective regulation of the private sector. Policy decisions should be based on appropriate "local" evidence in order to establish a pro-poor balance, among sub-sectors, such as between hospital and primary care, between urban and rural health services, and between basic care that helps many and costly specialized care that benefits a few. All of the case studies presented here entailed approaches designed to target and reduce these barriers, and most showed through monitoring and evaluation steps that they were pro-poor.

Financial barriers are especially significant where health systems rely on user fees at the time of service and where risk-pooling and pre-payment schemes have not been established. Not only do the direct costs of health care deter many sick people from seeking care, but other costs such as transport and food are important barriers to access, as are opportunity costs (e.g., income lost while seeking care or assisting a family member.) The Asia Pacific region has the highest percentage of out-of-pocket payment for health services of any of the WHO regions, and the reduction of this barrier is a regional priority for WHO. Three of the cases describe different approaches to targeting financial assistance to poorer households.

Geographical barriers result from the concentration of health facilities and health workers in urban areas and in areas with adequate transport. The poor and disadvantaged tend to live in the least-served areas, which also suffer the worst environmental conditions. Health workers generally prefer urban, higher income settings where there are more opportunities for them and their families. The remoteness of some areas remains a barrier even in some better-off countries, and the cost of reaching such populations with adequate care can be quite high.

Socio-cultural barriers may be based on social status or a consequence of the poverty and powerlessness associated with lower status, including ethnicity, gender and other social factors. Minority groups often have language and cultural differences from the majority population, including health workers, which constitutes a barrier to seeking or receiving adequate care. Gender is frequently a determinant of access to care in many settings, with women and girls receiving insufficient or delayed services more often than men or boys.

Poor responsiveness of the health system can be a problem, even where health facilities are available. Compared to complaints by those from better-off localities, complaints by the poor and disadvantaged are less likely to be heard and acted on. Common issues include inconvenient location of health facilities or working hours, rude or abusive health workers, more frequent problems in maintaining adequate stocks of medicines, and missing or malfunctioning equipment. Several of the cases presented here show how more resources were focused on specific diseases or environmental factors that especially affect the poor. Several others increased or monitored the resources allocated to geographical areas having a high percentage of poor or ethnic minority households.

Country examples of how evidence was used to stimulate pro-poor health policy-making

A major goal of policy research is to achieve a systematic understanding of what, when, and how research should feed into the development of policy. Such an understanding of how research can contribute to pro-poor policies, and systems to put it into practice, could improve health as well as development outcomes.

Most governments in the Western Pacific Region already have explicit pro-poor health policies in place, often as part of poverty reduction strategies, strategies for meeting the Millennium Development Goals, or in statements of national equity principles. Consequently, none of the case studies in this collection attempt to provide more evidence for the need to have pro-poor and pro-equity policies. Rather, they all focus on crucial details of why and how research was done and how the evidence was translated into policies and action.

Case studies are traditionally associated with business school, law school and social science, but can be used in any discipline to explore how issues and principles interact in real-world situations, and increasingly are being used to study development issues. Case studies can be a useful learning tool from which to draw lessons for adaptation and use in other contexts.

The countries represented in these case studies cover the spectrum of economic development, from the two with lowest per capita incomes, to the third wealthiest country in the Western Pacific Region, and the other five countries filling in the low-middle to high-middle income ranges. Their levels of health sector development and policy-making cover a similar wide range. All the cases identify and show evidence about specific equity issues. Some studies go into somewhat less detail about how the evidence was presented to policy-makers and how the policy process was influenced by the evidence, but enough is given to enable comparisons.

Guidelines for case study preparation (see Annex 1) were sent in advance to help ensure that the cases would be relevant to the health equity focus of the High-Level Meeting and to the agenda of examining the evidence-to-policy process. Most of the cases were prepared and presented through collaboration between a range of stakeholders, including local and international researchers, policy-makers, donors, and civil society organizations. The nine country cases presented at the High-Level Meeting (by meeting session) and compiled in this collection are:

Session 1: Health care financing

- *Health financing strategies to improve access to health services for the poor in Cambodia: from pilot to policy and action—a case study of Health Equity Funds.* Pro-poor health financing strategies developed in Cambodia in the 1990s led from user fees to contracting. The case examines steps taken to improve equity in health financing that culminated in the wide use of health equity funds (HEF).
- *Research, intervention design and policy implementation of the New Rural Cooperative Medical Scheme in Shandong, China.* This paper describes research and policy-making about adjusting the premium, subsidy, and benefit package at county level for the national insurance system for rural households, the New Cooperative Medical Services (NCMS) scheme.
- *Health Care Fund for the Poor in Viet Nam: how evidence and politics came together.* This paper is an overview of the evolution of the national health insurance scheme and examines how an effective and efficient way of subsidizing membership for the poor was devised, evaluated, and became official policy.

Session 2: Primary health care

- *Scaling up primary health care in the Lao People's Democratic Republic using evidence from a long-term primary health care development project.* This is a case study of a community-based, non-governmental organization (NGO)-sponsored project and how the results were disseminated and partially replicated. It includes an analysis of the roles of large donors and NGOs in policy decisions.
- *Promoting health equity: evidence, policy and action—the New Zealand experience.* This study described research into health problems of the Māori population and how they were effectively targeted by interventions to improve community-based primary health care services and housing conditions.

Session 3: Communicable diseases

- *The development and targeting of malaria control interventions for populations in high transmission areas of Cambodia: the influence of research on policy and practice.* This paper describes how field surveys resulted in operational changes in how malaria treatment is provided, and how insecticide-treated bednets are subsidized and targeted.
- *Public-Private Mix DOTS: a strategy to engage all health care providers in tuberculosis control and significantly increase access to DOTS services in the Philippines.* This paper discusses why and how private providers were incorporated into the national tuberculosis control programme, based on research that suggested the public sector alone could not achieve targets.

Session 4: Health systems

- *Geographic equity in distribution of scarce dialysis resources in Malaysia.* This research compares the provincial concentration of public, charitable, and private resources and determines that public funds subsidize the poor more than the well-off.
- *Promoting health equity through capacity building of primary health care workers in Mongolia.* This case documents how external resources were not used effectively to support rural health services, which led to a change in strategy for in-service training of mid-level staff by developing a local fellowship programme.

How evidence was used for policy-making in the cases

Previous research has identified factors that encourage good policy-making in terms of the relevance, effectiveness, efficiency, and timeliness of policies. The country cases in this collection illustrate several different types of policy impact. The small sample and many variables do not support a rigorous analysis, but factors in each case can be highlighted with the degree of uptake of evidence used as a measure of impact.

Overall, research evidence was used to make a concrete change in policy at some level in seven of the nine cases. However, variations are observed across countries. The use of evidence ranges from rapid adoption as national policy, to changes in how existing policy was implemented, to very slow or no uptake. In Malaysia, for example, policy change did not result, because it was not an intended outcome of the research.

In Viet Nam, evidence was used to support a new central government health financing policy and guide development of a programme that established a system of subsidized health insurance cards for the poor. The policy decision does not rigidly spell out details, leaving some to be resolved by future research and planning.

In the Philippines, the evidence was used to show a need for a public-private partnership strategy, and later that the pilots of that approach were effective and should be replicated. In China, evidence convinced policy-makers to allow the use of Medical Assistance Funds to pay NCMS insurance premiums for the poor. Most recommendations were accepted and implemented at local level. In Cambodia, evidence that health equity funds were efficient and equitable resulted in acceptance and replication, but although HEFs are recognized as a tool for achieving equity and poverty reduction, they have not become an official financing policy.

Several cases show how evidence led to policy changes aiming to improve the implementation of existing programmes. In China, the evidence informed the recommendations to revise NCMS subsidies and to add benefits at the county level. In Cambodia evidence resulted in a decision to extend the geographical eligibility for free bednets and to rely on village workers to distribute antimalarial drugs in the least accessible areas, leaving the social marketing programme to focus on other endemic areas. In Mongolia, the evidence supported a shift in training policy from overseas fellowships to local fellowships.

In several cases, research was used to verify that an intervention was pro-poor. In Malaysia, for example, the geographical distribution of dialysis facilities was monitored over time, confirming that there was a relative increase in the use of government facilities. Research on equity funds in Cambodia verified that subsidies were targeted accurately and efficiently. The uptake of health care cards was monitored in Viet Nam in order to identify operational problems.

In some cases, the evidence was not immediately adopted in policy or action. In the Lao People's Democratic Republic, the rural project's community-based strategy was not replicated for several years, partly because evidence of the project's success was not considered to be strong, and because policy-making favoured large-scale, top-down health development projects. In China the recommendation to increase individual premiums was not immediately acted on in two of the three counties because local managers were reluctant to increase premiums, which they feared would result in lower NCMS enrolment. In the Philippines, several elements of the Comprehensive and Unified Policy for TB Control were not implemented, for lack of financing and support.

Contemporary models of the research-to-policy process

Policy-making is not linear and is rarely a unique or explicit set of decisions, but evolves through multiple interactions and different sources of knowledge, usually engaging a range of actors and stakeholders. Especially in the arena of health policy and equity, it is a multidimensional process that can entail iterations in the form of population surveys, pilot projects, evaluations, welfare analysis, and other complementary studies. There may be no clear distinction between researchers and policy-makers, often because of the small pool of concerned stakeholders and limited resources. Finally, production of knowledge is not always limited to a set of specific findings, because of time lags in research and new policy issues being raised through research in other countries.

Reflecting this understanding of policy-making, the relationship between research and policy is also no longer thought of as a linear or purely rational process in which research findings are shifted from the 'research sphere' over to the 'policy sphere', where they then have some impact on policy-makers' decisions.

The "Policy Wheel" (Figure 1) as developed by Dr. Don Matheson and colleagues in New Zealand depicts the iterative and continuous nature of this process. It serves as a guide for each of the policy development stages, from problem assessment to policy change and implementation.

The crucial question engaging policy researchers is: why are some ideas that circulate in the research–policy arena picked up and acted on, while others are ignored and disappear? Several useful frameworks or models have been used to evaluate the process through which research leads to policy and action. None of these has as yet attempted to be predictive in the sense that weights can be given to factors and the probability of policy uptake then calculated. It can be reasonably said that all plausible models are currently of equal precision and utility, varying chiefly in the definition of the factors rather than on their relative importance, which are not yet known empirically.

These models have helped identify critical factors associated with effective use of high-quality evidence. Most are based on experience from industrialized countries, however, and the diversity of cultural, economic, and political contexts in the less developed countries makes it difficult to draw valid generalizations and lessons from them. In addition, international

Figure 1: The Policy Wheel

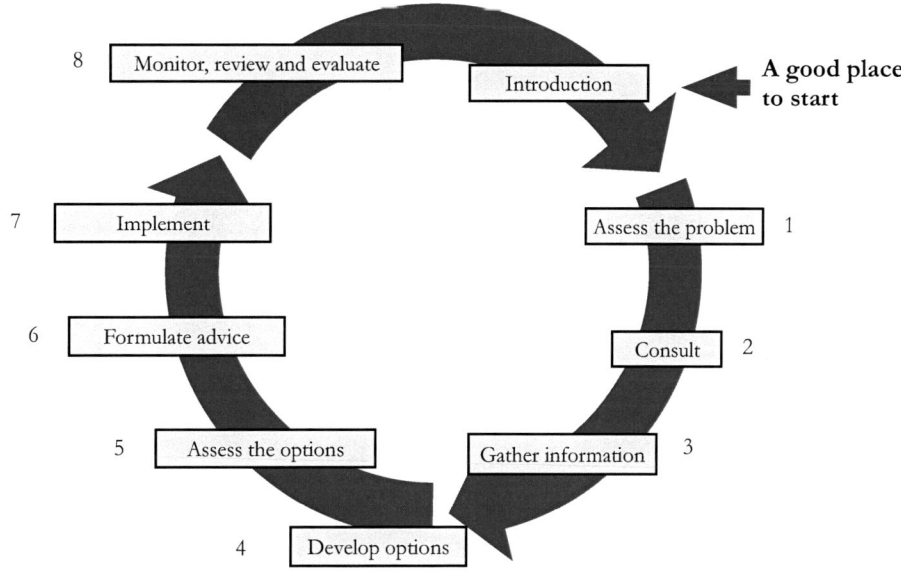

actors continue to exert much influence on health research and policy processes in developing countries. Nevertheless, some observations on the research-to-policy process can be made.

Most models and frameworks propose common factors which determine the influence of evidence on policy: 1) the context in which the policy and evidence are situated; 2) the content, timeliness, and credibility of the evidence; and 3) actors and the interaction between them, to which can be added the effect of external influences. These frameworks can illuminate significant aspects of the case studies presented in this book. Some models discussed at the High-Level Meeting are summarized here:

1. The RAPID Framework[2] (Figure 2) is based on a comparative analysis of 50 cases on the research-to-policy process in the international development field. Research uptake is seen as a function of the interaction of context, evidence, and links. External influences also bear on all of these.

2. A variation on the above model, the "4K framework"[3] was used by researchers in one of the case studies presented here ("Health financing strategies to improve access to health services for the poor in Cambodia: from pilot to policy and action—A case study of Health Equity Funds"). The 4K framework describes four stages: Stage 1 of exploitation of existing knowledge; Stage 2 of creating of new knowledge or innovation; Stage 3 of disseminating the new knowledge or evidence brokering; and Stage 4 of adopting and using the new knowledge. Each stage was analysed by determinants of context, content and actors, similar to those of the RAPID model.

3. A framework by Lavis et al.[4] overlaps with the RAPID framework's context and linkages or the 4K framework's context and actors. Four alternative models of the demand for and use of research evidence are described, as stemming from 1) a "push" by research producers or purveyors, 2) a "pull" by research users, 3) an "exchange" between single groups of research producers and users, or 4) "integrated" efforts that involve such knowledge translation platforms as the Evidence-Informed Policy Network (EVIPNet).

Figure 2: The RAPID Framework: Context, Evidence and Links

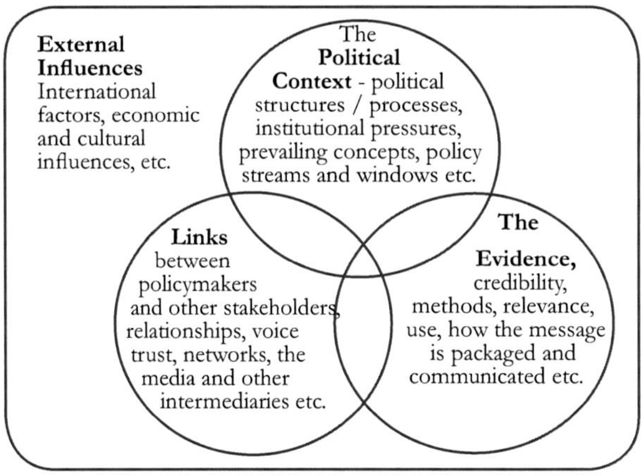

Source: Court and Young 2002.

Lessons from the processes described in country case studies

Only a few of the cases here illustrate the policy process in its entirety. Instead, most focus on one or more phases or stages of the overall process. The China case study describes a fairly thorough but narrowly focused assessment of problems with the NCMS, but did not discuss wider issues of health equity and financing. The Cambodia and Viet Nam financing reforms were done in the context of fairly comprehensive evaluations of equity and financing, but these were the background to the HEF and Health Care Fund for the Poor (HCFP) strategies and not direct parts of the policy process. A more rigorous approach to problem assessment can be made, as shown in a recent description[5] of equity policy in South Africa. Most of the cases also did not include in significant detail steps 4 and 5 of the policy wheel, in which options are developed and evaluated. The Cambodia financing study comes the closest but, in actuality, the health equity funds were introduced as a complement to other financing modes and did not replace the existing modes. Most of the cases do describe the evaluation and consultation steps in the process fairly thoroughly, in part because the instructions for case preparation stressed this.

The nine cases in this collection are diverse but also have elements in common. The uptake of evidence by policy-makers can be seen as the outcome of the research-to-policy process, or as a dependent variable. Independent variables can be described in terms of factors that map on to the *context, evidence, links, and external influences,* used in the RAPID model and others.

The case studies can be compared using the following expanded categories, which are discussed below, and also summarized in Table 1 on page 20:

1. Context (including external influences)
    a. The reasons the research was carried out
    b. The primary focus of the polic(ies) the case study influenced
    c. Specific access barrier or equity issue and the type of equity analysis used in generating the evidence
2. Evidence (or content)
    a. The type of research done and the quality of evidence produced
    b. Whether the research evidence provided an operational solution to a problem
3. Links and actors (including external influences)
    a. The types of collaboration between researchers and policy-makers
    b. Stakeholder interactions that affect the uptake of research for policy.

1. Context

Context covers a number of important enabling factors[6] that affect the degree to which research has an impact on policy. It includes health and equity status, prevailing opinions (local and from other countries), existing policy commitments, related discourse among policy-makers, and the extent of demand for new ideas by policy-makers and society generally ("pull" factors). The existence and nature of prior research on a given policy issue is another important context factor. These contextual influences are summarized in Table 1 on page 20.

Context (a): Why was the research done?

Because they were deliberately selected as such, there was a commitment to improving equity in all the countries and case studies. Individual research goals may have been determined by social and political environment, the existing health system situation and capacity, and the demand for policy change. The latter factor is relevant to the *push /pull/ exchange/ integrated* model of Lavis *et al.*, and also to the linkages between stakeholders.

In all of the cases, *prior evidence of the lack of equity from pre-existing research* was an important stimulus for finding effective interventions. The processes that were described in Cambodia and Viet Nam made extensive use of studies that had found evidence of unequal provision and uptake of public subsidies and differentials in health status. Such evidence also existed in China. The full cost of kidney dialysis treatment was known to be unaffordable for many Malaysians, and the disadvantaged status of Māori in New Zealand had been thoroughly documented. Rural Mongolians were known to be disadvantaged in terms of disease incidence and availability of health services, as were people in a remote province in the Lao People's Democratic Republic. It was also found that tuberculosis sufferers in the Philippines are much poorer than average, as are malaria victims in hyperendemic areas of Cambodia.

Commitment to improving equity and the current policies that affect it was another main reason for the research described in several case studies. Evidence of worsening health conditions and international scrutiny of China's health system led to more attention by the central government focused on equity issues and especially rural health care. The low reimbursement rates were based on political considerations because leaders needed to be seen as doing something about health, and a small benefit package is easily delivered to a large population while keeping the premium low. The goal of the research was to improve the NCMS in terms of equity, quality, and efficiency using evidence-based interventions. The China case is an example of research being *pulled* by demand (by national priorities and from a multi-country policy research project), and it also involved considerable *exchange* between researchers and policy-makers.

The Cambodia study of health equity funds described how research and pilot project evaluations established HEFs as an accepted health financing strategy. Evidence showing that adequate public health services could not be provided free of charge for all population groups prompted the Ministry of Health to identify and test alternative financing strategies, including user fees with exemptions, contracting, health equity funds and community-based health insurance. The policy process relied heavily on research on interventions that took place over nearly a decade.

The Viet Nam study documents the evolution of pro-poor national health financing policies in response to deterioration in equity following the transition to a free market system. User fees were introduced in 1989 in response to a shortfall in funding for the health system. An overall pro-poor policy and goal of universal insurance coverage had been stated clearly in policy documents, and a prevention-oriented health system was functional. There were mechanisms in place for interacting with the poor locally, and the Viet Nam Health Insurance Agency was in favor of expanding coverage by means of subsidies. In both Viet Nam and Cambodia, the need to attack the causes of poverty and the strong support of donors facilitated the research.

In Mongolia, rural-urban migration deprived the rural areas of amenities as well as trained human resources. Evaluations of the existing training strategy found that it was not meeting the needs of rural areas, and identified potential benefits of a local fellowship programme. This strategy was tested and accepted as a component of health human resource policy.

To monitor implementation of existing policy: A secondary purpose of the research in Viet Nam was to monitor poverty reduction effects of the evolving health financing policy and whether the health cards were targeted accurately. The research described in the Malaysia case study was intended to verify that the existing policy of pro-poor and pro-rural public health provision was being followed in practice. The Philippines PPMD project, Cambodia malaria interventions, and Cambodia HEF development relied heavily on evaluations of pilot projects to guide policy development or change. The Mongolia case study describes a preliminary assessment of the new local fellowship training program.

To provide support and guidance for disease control programmes was the principal aim of the Cambodia malaria case study, which was specifically aimed at improving the efficiency and effectiveness of preventive and curative interventions implemented under the National Malaria Programme. The Philippines PPMD study focused on combating tuberculosis by broadening the provider base for the existing TB control programme.

To inform or refine donor assistance was another secondary reason for several studies. The Cambodia health financing study showed that Health Equity Funds are an effective and efficient way to target donor funding at the poor. The Mongolia study demonstrated that the shift in WHO funding to local fellowships was effective in reaching a larger number of rural workers, should be expanded, and also has attracted other potential donors. The Lao People's Democratic Republic study described how evidence was intended to encourage the Government and donors to fund the expansion of the community-oriented primary health care strategy. The Cambodia malaria case study and the Philippines PPMD studies were used to justify continued funding from the Global Fund and other donors.

Context (b): What specific equity objectives were addressed in the studies?

Poverty reduction as a national policy goal was the focus of several country cases. The China NCMS case involved a key element of the national poverty reduction strategy. As in Mongolia and Viet Nam, China's economic transition has resulted in rural areas becoming relatively disadvantaged. Implementation of the NCMS is decentralized and the research and policy work was specific to six counties in two provinces, but it is likely that national policy will be revised on the basis of these studies.

The Viet Nam case describes the steps that led to an official decision to subsidize social health insurance as part of the national poverty reduction strategy. This work was carried out on the national level, with attention given to differences between provinces in their ability to finance the scheme.

Equity and poverty were intensively researched in Cambodia, and the health sector plays an important role in the poverty reduction strategy. The research described in the case study confirmed that health equity funds can reduce out-of-pocket expenditures in most situations. HEFs are mentioned as a possible poverty reduction strategy in national plans, and government funds have been allocated to HEFs, but they do not yet have formal status in national policy.

Reducing urban-rural inequality as a national policy goal was implicit in the China case, since the NCMS is a national programme to benefit rural households. The rural population was found to spend a higher proportion of incomes on health and receive less public subsidy than urban residents. The NCMS is intended to both assure access to all rural residents via near-universal insurance coverage, and to revive the public health care in rural areas by channeling provincial and local subsidies to public health facilities.

Inequality is addressed in the Malaysia case through research confirming that the national pro-rural and pro-poor policy of subsidizing health services was being maintained. The methodology used measured geographical equity of dialysis as a proxy for income or vertical equity.

The Mongolia case was a response to a shortage of rural health workers, where evidence generated guided the design of a cost-effective programme of local long-term training. The new local training strategy is implemented at the national level.

The primary health care development programme described in the Lao People's Democratic Republic case improved access to health services in a remote rural province. The project was tailored to needs of local people, but many of the same conditions are found in other rural areas. The national health strategy prioritizes the development of primary health care in rural areas, but the case showed that community-based approaches are not always considered to be replicable.

Reducing morbidity from specific poverty-related diseases and achieving MDG targets was the goal of the Philippines PPMD project, launched in order to improve TB case detection rates. Similarly, the Cambodia malaria studies came about in response to hyperendemicity and high mortality from malaria in several areas of the country. Malaria incidence in the three lowest income quintiles was several times more than in the two highest ones.

Engaging and monitoring the non-state (private and NGO) sector was another policy goal of the Philippines PPMD Directly-Observed Treatment Short-Course (DOTS) strategy. The private sector was found to be an important TB service provider, but the quality of treatment was often low. Participation of private providers opened ways for local partnerships, NGOs and corporations to become directly involved in TB control, and also local governments as the payers in the devolved health system.

The aim of the Malaysia case was to determine if the rapid growth of private and charitable dialysis services was affecting the overall pro-poor policy in health service provision. The private sector was found to concentrate dialysis centres in economically developed states where patients could afford to pay. While the publicly provided share of dialysis has decreased, the public sector still focuses on the poorer states but the NGO sector surprisingly parallels the private sector in locating dialysis centres.

The Lao People's Democratic Republic case illustrates collaboration between an NGO and the provincial health department in the development of a community-based primary health care programme, but the Ministry of Health gives more priority to large-scale, top-down, donor-funded health development projects. In contrast, the New Zealand case describes policy changes that utilized the effective role of Primary Health Organizations, non-governmental units that specifically focus on the health needs of local communities.

Context (c): Which access barriers were addressed in the country cases?

Financial barriers to access to health services were the focus of five country cases. Despite the continuous development of pro-poor health policies in Viet Nam, including mandated exemptions and subsidized health insurance, private expenditure and out-of-pocket payments remained high. Limited funding for subsidies and lack of strong commitment from local governments compounded the problem of unaffordability of public services. In response, the government introduced the Health Care Fund for the Poor, which provides health insurance subsidies financed from the central budget.

The Cambodia Health Equity Funds case addressed the problem of catastrophic payments directly by introducing local financing schemes that cover user fees at hospitals for the poor. A demographic survey in 1999 found that the poor had much lower use of health services than the rich, suffered more illness, and spent a much higher proportion of household income on health care.

The China study found that high hospital co-payments were a barrier to utilization, but also that most non-poor people could afford to pay more than the current NCMS premium. Evidence from a baseline household survey guided recommendations for adjusting NCMS premium and benefits and for using a separate fund to subsidize insurance premiums for the poor.

In the Philippines, TB is largely a disease of the poor and TB drugs are expensive. The case describes a strategy for using private providers to increase coverage of free DOTS diagnosis and treatment. In Malaysia, free public provision of kidney dialysis was introduced, to overcome the potentially catastrophic costs of this treatment. The case verifies that public sector provision is still pro-poor.

Overcoming geographical barriers to access was a major focus of the Lao People's Democratic Republic case, where a highly decentralized approach succeeded in providing services to a remote mountainous area. In Cambodia, malaria is endemic in remote forested areas, and baseline research was used to develop a programme of village malaria workers to diagnose and treat suspected cases in these areas. Other evidence led to expanded free bednet distribution in those areas. An assessment in the Philippines showed that DOTS coverage was inadequate in some of the largest urban areas. Establishment of private sector DOTS units in underserved areas helped to increase the national case detection rate by 18%.

Barriers caused by social exclusion are highlighted by the New Zealand case, which describes how the Māori population was shown to have worse health outcomes than other groups, largely due to discrimination and exclusion. A new primary health care programme was designed to overcome these barriers, complemented by a targeted, multisectoral, housing improvement programme. The needs of specific social groups were also addressed by the Cambodia malaria interventions since the hyperendemic forested areas are largely populated by ethnic minorities.

Social exclusion is closely tied to the problem of *health system unresponsiveness*. The primary health care strategy described in the Lao People's Democratic Republic case included addressing the needs of ethnic minorities using health workers who spoke their languages and were sensitive to their beliefs and customs, and provided outreach services to communities with difficult access to fixed services. Inability to stem the outflow of rural health workers in Mongolia was one of the reasons for persistent high infant and child mortality and morbidity rates. The failure of the official exemption systems that led to reforms in Cambodia and Viet Nam is another example of how health systems do not respond to the needs of the poor.

2. Evidence and communication

Analysis of standards in health policy research, especially that related to equity, is at an early stage of development. Various "hierarchy of evidence" systems have been described. Figure 3 shows one such typology of research evidence. In general, higher-level analysis and systematic reviews are considered superior forms of evidence than case studies.[7]

Figure 3: Hierarchy of evidence: ranking of research evidence evaluating health care interventions

	Effectiveness	Appropriateness	Feasibility
Excellent	• Systematic Review • Multi-centre studies	• Systematic Review • Multi-centre studies	• Systematic Review • Multi-centre studies
Good	• RCT • Observational studies	• RCT • Observational studies • Interpretative studies	• RCT • Observational studies • Interpretative studies
Fair	• Uncontrolled trials with dramatic results • Before and after studies • Non-randomized controlled trials	• Descriptive studies • Focus groups	• Descriptive studies • Action research • Before and after studies • Focus groups
Poor	• Descriptive studies • Case studies • Expert opinion • Studies of poor methodological quality	• Expert opinion • Case studies • Studies of poor methodological quality	• Expert opinion • Case studies • Studies of poor methodological quality

Source: Evans D. 2003.

However, classifications such as the above and others[8] are not very relevant to equity policy development and public health interventions, where tools such as double-blind trials are not generally feasible. Case studies are usually more common than most of the other, stronger forms of evidence. Much can be learned from well done case studies, and especially from reviews based on several case studies in the context of a single country.

The influence of research on policy is much increased if it has topical relevance and operational usefulness. The most important factors enabling uptake of research evidence were found by Court and Young to be whether the evidence was presented effectively as a practical solution to a problem and was credible in terms of research approach. A "knowledge pyramid"[9] with actionable messages at the apex is applicable to equity policy.

Figure 4: Knowledge pyramid

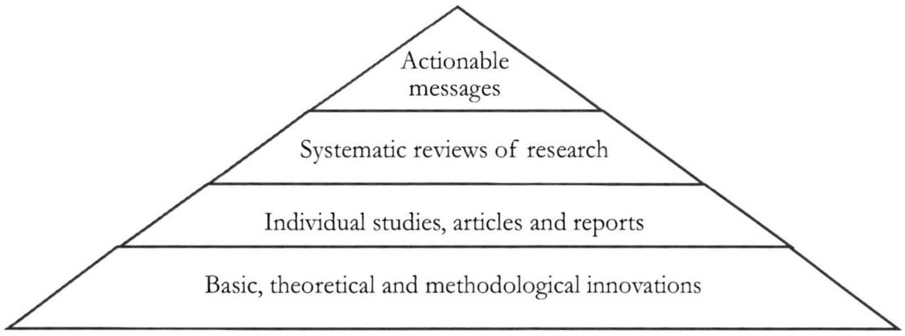

```
              /\
             /  \
            / Actionable \
           /  messages  \
          /--------------\
         / Systematic reviews of research \
        /----------------------------------\
       / Individual studies, articles and reports \
      /--------------------------------------------\
     / Basic, theoretical and methodological innovations \
    /------------------------------------------------------\
```

Source: Lavis et. al 2006.

Actionable messages should ideally be based on entire bodies of research knowledge, not just individual studies, and stakeholders should try to achieve consensus on the messages that are conveyed. An optimum strategy may be to focus knowledge-transfer efforts at the apex of the knowledge pyramid using actionable messages, while continuing to build a solid knowledge base. The various types of evidence generated in the nine cases, and their operational usefulness, are summarized in Table 1 on page 20.

Evidence and communication (a): What kinds of research methods and evidence were used in the cases?

Various types of evidence were generated by the research discussed in the country cases. A range of methodological approaches was taken in response to the challenge of assessing equity issues. There was also variation in the intensity of the research and the resources required. These in turn affected the overall time frame of the research-to-policy process.

Baseline studies were the foundation of much of the evidence used in the China policy development process. Townships and counties were selected randomly for three research activities, a health survey of 3,339 households, an organizational analysis, and focus group discussions. A 2003 national survey also provided evidence of the high financial burden from hospital co-payments, finding that hospital costs were high and reimbursements low.

Baseline surveys also underpinned the intervention trials in the case related to the Cambodia malaria programme, the Mongolia rural human resource case, and the New Zealand primary health care case. In the last, it was shown that Māori people have poorer access than other groups to health services, poorer quality of care within the health system and worse health outcomes for most disease groups. In Viet Nam, equity was researched in depth through a participatory poverty assessment that found that user fees at hospitals imposed a high financial burden on poor households, and through two living standards measurement surveys that showed that the poor utilize services less than the rich and capture a smaller share of public subsidies. The HCFP policy process was guided by several studies of the new financing policies, including some based on large validated survey datasets and done by reputed local and foreign researchers. The evidence and policy recommendations took place over a period of 8 to 12 years, with evaluations at several stages of the development process. The finding of significantly higher utilization of public health services by insurance beneficiaries supported universal health insurance and identified shortcomings in existing financing arrangements, culminating in Decision 139 to increase insurance benefits, coverage, and central government funding.

The Cambodia HEF case similarly used evidence from prior health financing interventions as well as several studies of at least twenty HEF pilot projects. Evidence was considered reliable, and showed that HEFs helped reduce financial barriers to access to timely and needed care for poor patients, while maintaining the income of public health facilities. The data required significant analysis and interpretation since it consisted of a large number of studies.

Concrete proposals for policy changes or interventions were derived from the research evidence in all of these cases. The evidence was considered to be credible because of the professional status of the researchers and the apparent validity of the data.

Pilot interventions and their evaluations were used to generate credible evidence in some of the case studies. This evidence tends to be highly focused and easy to understand, which may explain why these types of analyses have resulted in policy changes relatively quickly. This was true of the pilot village malaria worker interventions in Cambodia, where an evaluation demonstrated that it was cost-effective enough to be scaled up. In contrast, the other element of the Cambodia malaria case, a malariometric survey of sample communities, did not involve a pilot, but by showing that malaria risk outside the forest areas was higher than had been previously believed, it led directly to a change in the bednet distribution coverage area and reallocation of programme resources. In the Philippines case, analysis of pilots at several sites showed that PPMD was effective and recommended that it should be scaled up. Assessment of the Mongolia Local Fellowship Training Programme showed that the strategy was widely accepted by health workers and other stakeholders, and was successful in that all local training fellows returned to their place of work and some initiated new community health programmes.

The Lao People's Democratic Republic case was based on evaluations of each of the four phases of the project. Evaluations were built into the project and were carried out by qualified researchers, but in the view of some policy-makers the lack of an initial baseline survey was a weakness. The replicability of the project was also questioned by policy-makers.

Evidence and communication (b): Was a practical solution to an operational problem recommended?

Operational recommendations were not the only goal of the research in some cases. Several types of policy recommendation came from the research evidence.

In China, specific recommendations on the need to increase premiums and benefits were communicated to county-level managers, as well as a proposal to use the Medical Assistance Fund to pay NCMS premiums for the poor. The Cambodia malaria studies focused on operational problems and offered detailed recommendations for resolving them. The Cambodia health financing reforms and Health Equity Fund evaluations produced a concrete recommendation that the Ministry of Economy and Finance should allocate a budget for these decentralized funds, which included basic policy guidelines for the HEF mechanism, but left some policy issues unresolved, awaiting further research. This was true in New Zealand as well, where it was recommended that community-run primary health care providers be given latitude to deal with local health issues. Another set of studies identified specific housing issues, and did make recommendations to correct the observed problems.

In the Philippines case, since the strategy of involving the private sector was developed and piloted first and then evaluated, the analysis resulted only in a recommendation that the approach should be officially adopted by the Department of Health. Similarly in Mongolia, the strategy of local fellowship training was developed independently, with subsequent research verifying that it was effective. This basically happened in the case of health cards for the poor in Viet Nam as well. Early research found a need to assist the poor, and several approaches were successively implemented and evaluated, leading to refinements and the eventual development of the HCFP policy.

The Malaysia case study was a one-off evaluation made after a long process of development of dialysis services, with the actual research completed in a short time. It resulted in no new recommendations, other than continuing the existing policy because it was found that the government provision was still pro-poor even as the private and NGO sectors expanded their services.

The Lao People's Democratic Republic case study focuses on the recommendation that the primary health care approach and strategy tried in Sayaboury province should be scaled up. Details were made available about the successful project elements but the project was not replicated as the NGO had recommended, in part because some of the evidence was felt to be unconvincing, but also because it was thought that the presence of a highly skilled expatriate adviser was essential to its success and could not be replicated.

3. Links between stakeholders and the role of external influences

The nature of collaboration between researchers and policy-makers is considered to be a key determinant of the success of the overall evidence-to-policy process. This includes the quality of the links and feedback processes inherent to the process, some of which are described in the cases. Issues of trust, legitimacy, openness and formalization of networks are understood to be important, as is the role of "translation" of technical content into simple language and its effective communication. Often, intermediary organizations and networks influence formal policy guidance documents, which, in turn, influence officials. The RAPID framework emphasizes the importance of links through communities, networks and intermediaries (e.g. the media and lobbying groups) in effecting policy change. The linkage model of Lavis *et al.* highlights advantages of the "exchange" and "networked" processes.

Policy uptake has been found to be greatest if the research programme has a clear communication strategy from the start, and if the results are packaged in familiar concepts. It is often difficult to convince policy-makers of the value of more theoretical research if it is not clearly linked to policy applications. The sources and conveyors of information, the way new messages are packaged (e.g., couched in familiar or unfamiliar terms) and targeted can affect how policy documents are perceived and utilized. Continuous interaction leads to greater chances of successful communication than a simple or linear approach.

The cases illustrate various types of collaboration arrangements between stakeholders, as well as several variations in the way stakeholders collaborated. The details of who did the research, who funded the research, and which stakeholders were involved in disseminating the evidence and generating policy recommendations, are shown in Table 1. In addition to the researchers, the stakeholders included central and local health and finance authorities, NGOs that were concerned with specific health issues and/or communities, and donors or donor consortia. The researchers were from academic institutions, Government (executive and research branches), and consultants employed by donors.

Resistance to policy change and how to overcome it

Despite the existence of clear evidence, efforts to improve equity often challenge structures of social and economic power, leading to political resistance that can impede change. Bureaucratic factors, institutional pressures, and vested interests can also distort policies during implementation. The existence of a degree of openness and civil and political freedoms can sometimes effectively counter these other contextual factors. In several of the cases, the advantages of close collaboration were demonstrated clearly.

Stakeholders from the policy arena in the cases discussed here mainly include public health and finance officials, and to a lesser extent, civil society through NGOs. There is little mention of mass public support or opposition to policies. In these cases, resistance to policy change comes from specific vested interests or bureaucratic factors. Overcoming such opposition requires effective communication between researchers, policy-makers and other stakeholders. Two cases that describe positive policy outcomes—China and the Philippines— emphasize the importance of personal and group communication strategies. Other successful processes, such as in the Viet Nam and Cambodia HEF cases, rely more on formal policy dialogues between national counterparts and donors, and, in the New Zealand case, with civil society stakeholders.

In China, researchers accorded top priority to maintaining a formal relationship with policy-makers through the project, which facilitated good communication. All the stakeholders were included in designing the study. Policy-makers from several government departments were involved in designing the intervention packages and shared the responsibility for their implementation. Local-level policy-makers and managers discussed and evaluated the results in public meetings. Researchers provided continuing support to the policy-makers during the post-research phases. There was relatively little direct influence by donors; the project was monitored by WHO and other donors, and EVIPNet also participated. There was some resistance from policy-makers and managers, whose performance ratings could be affected if enrollments decreased due to higher individual premiums. On the other hand, there was little opposition to raising public (county) subsidies to NCMS, or to using a Medical Assistance Fund that is under different management and budget from the NCMS to subsidize premiums for the poor. In addition, the central government announced an increase in NCMS provincial subsidies.

In the Philippines case, there was initial opposition from the public health establishment to involving the private sector in TB control, but the successful pilot projects and a collegial research and policy atmosphere helped overcome this. The research was carried out by the Department of Health and WHO in collaboration with the major project implementer (PhilCAT). Personal contacts enhanced the exchange of information and policy discussions, and the lines between researchers, implementers, and policy-makers were not consistently fixed. The financial participation of the stakeholder PhilHealth to provide private physician reimbursement for TB outpatient treatment was also critical to the success of the PPMD.

International partners and donors and donor funding have a special role both in stimulating research and enabling research to have an impact on policy. For example, WHO technical inputs, and broad incentives such the Global Fund, the Millennium Development Goals (MDGs), and the poverty reduction strategy paper (PRSP) process, have had substantial impacts.

In Viet Nam, government at all levels was concerned about the affordability of insurance premiums by the poor, but the Ministry of Finance was reluctant to increase health spending by subsidizing the poor through the insurance scheme. Ministry of Health policy researchers used evidence from World Bank, Asian Development Bank, and WHO studies to formulate recommendations, with close contact between all stakeholders maintained through the process.

In addition, research was funded and guided by the major donors in several cases. The Cambodia malaria case was based on donor-funded research, as was the development of the local fellowship scheme in Mongolia. In the Mongolia case, there was little opposition, perhaps because continuing the overseas fellowships would have benefited relatively few people. The Sector-Wide Approach used in Cambodia provided an *exchange* environment, to use the terminology of the model developed by Lavis *et al.*, in which donors to the health sector were able to coordinate their inputs into equity research and pilot financing reforms. Evaluations by credible researchers and organizations were widely disseminated. Formal and informal meetings, workshops, conferences and study tours helped to inform policy-makers. There was little opposition to the expansion because the HEFs are seen as complementary to contracting, currently the most important financing scheme. Being locally generated, HEFs enjoyed ownership among health policy-makers and were easy to understand and implement, without threatening the interests of any stakeholder. Community-based insurance are seen as having some advantages, but have had relatively little support.

Table 1: An overview of the nine country cases

Case	Context	Evidence and its dissemination	Linkages and external influences	Policy outcome
Health financing strategies to improve access to health services for the poor in Cambodia: from pilot to policy and action—A case study of Health Equity Funds	Strong government equity commitment; previous financing reforms, extensive existing research, many HEF pilots.	Many pilots were evaluated; HEFs are shown to be efficient. Operationally useful findings.	Sector-wide approach, availability of donor and NGO funding for research and pilots. Ministry of Health and academic researchers involved.	HEFs have been widely adopted but are not yet official policy.
Research, intervention design and policy implementation of the New Rural Cooperative Medical Scheme in Shandong, China	Need to improve NCMS; focus on rural areas; multinational research project.	Evidence considered sound. Many meetings and workshops to discuss and develop feasible interventions.	Participation of EVIPNet and support from key donors.	Pilot interventions evaluated. Premium, benefit, Medical Assistance Fund policies were changed.
Health Care Fund for the Poor in Viet Nam: how evidence and politics came together	Strong equity commitment; previous financing reforms and evaluations, Ministry of Finance supports increasing subsidy, functioning PHC and identification of poor.	Quality research over several years in health financing. Continuous policy dialogue on health insurance.	Availability of donor funding for research. Ministry of Health and academic researchers involved. Ministry of Finance got good evidence to increase financing.	Decision 139 was enacted at Prime Ministerial level. Beneficiary identification is being steadily improved.
Scaling up primary health care in the Lao People's Democratic Republic using evidence from a long-term primary health care development project	Weak emphasis on PHC in Master Plan; large "top-down" projects receive Ministry of Health attention; NGOs have little influence.	Some evidence was considered weak. Reliance on documents to disseminate evidence.	Major project donor support stopped. Replication considered difficult.	There was acceptance in principle but dissemination has been slow

(Table 1 continued on next page)

In New Zealand and Malaysia, research units within the Ministry of Health played a major role in the entire process In the New Zealand case, a research unit in the Ministry of Health developed the evidence used in the primary health care intervention for Māori health, and an intersectoral collaboration that benefited both ministries led to the housing intervention. The Malaysia country case was also developed by a research unit within the Health Ministry. In the Lao People's Democratic Republic case, the research was initiated and funded by the NGO and bilateral donor that implemented the project. The provincial health office participated in the research.

(Table 1 continued)

Case	Context	Evidence and its dissemination	Linkages and external influences	Policy outcome
Promoting health equity: evidence, policy and action—The New Zealand experience	Policy commitment to remove inequalities; existing research	Careful studies considered valid evidence. Operational recommendations made.	Community organizations played large role. Housing Ministry worked with Ministry of Health.	Existing policies reinforced, successful interventions made.
The development and targeting of malaria control interventions for populations in high transmission areas of Cambodia: the influence of research on policy and practice	Malaria programme needed to combat fake drugs and poor access to health services in remote areas; existing programmes for bednet distribution.	Strong evidence that village malaria workers provided effective diagnosis and treatment and of wider malaria endemicity than assumed.	Ministry of Health and other stakeholders kept informed; Ministry of Health had to be convinced to use malaria volunteers; high-level dissemination event of pilot results.	Scaled up village malaria workers with Global Fund support. Bednet distribution strategy was changed.
Public-private mix DOTS: a strategy to engage all health care providers in tuberculosis control and significantly increase access to DOTS services in the Philippines	Nearly half of TB cases treated in private sector, but not always properly. Insurance reimbursement is available to private physicians.	Pilot projects were successful. Case detection increased significantly after scale-up.	Close contact between Department of Health researchers and NGO implementers. Global Fund supported expansion.	The Public-Private Strategy was adopted and has been scaled up.
Geographic equity in distribution of scarce dialysis resources in Malaysia	Pro-rural, pro-poor policy; growth of private and NGO sector, increasing national wealth.	Rural/urban was used as a proxy for income.	Ministry of Health did research and also was main client.	No change because a satisfactory pro-poor public subsidy was demonstrated.
Promoting health equity through capacity building of primary health care workers in Mongolia	Depletion of rural health workers was thought to be affecting rural health status.	Overseas Fellowship Study found problems which suggested that better results could be obtained from local training.	WHO involvement was important.	Local training strategy was accepted and other donors may participate.

Conclusions and future agenda

With minor exceptions, the cases from the Western Pacific Region presented at the High-Level Meeting on Promoting Health Equity: Evidence, Policy and Action were consistent with current models of the research-to-policy process. Table 1 summarizes the cases, showing the policy outcome alongside the significant factors of context, evidence and dissemination, and the relevant links and external influences, as used in contemporary models of the evidence-to-policy process.

Best use of the evidence for policy development was made in cases where the research was considered thorough and credible. A participatory approach that involved policy-makers and researchers, and a careful communication strategy also facilitated the use of evidence.

These two factors were especially clearly illustrated in the cases of the Cambodia HEF, the Viet Nam Health Care Fund for the Poor, and the China NCMS. In Cambodia, for example, the political environment was conducive, with openness and support for innovations, and the evidence was generated and communicated in a credible and timely manner, thanks in part to the sector-wide approach used there. In the Lao People's Democratic Republic case, the evidence was not as convincing, and rather than a collaborative environment, there was some resistance to the replication of the primary health care pilot project and more priority given to large-scale donor projects. In the Philippines PPMD case, the participatory and collaborative environment was perhaps as important as the actual evidence of project success. In New Zealand, policy changes followed a planned process (as described in the Policy Wheel), which ensured that the evidence was strong and all stakeholders were actively involved.

The experiences of eight countries as shown in these cases reveal many insights into how the policy development process works and how it can be improved. In the future, it may be possible to direct new case studies toward examining some specific questions. These include:

a. How can contexts be categorized and how best can stakeholders operate to influence policy in these different contexts? How do research–policy processes work in situations with democratic deficits? What can realistically be done to improve the context for the use of research in policy-making and practice?
b. Evidence: In this domain, there is still need for work on two main sets of issues. First, regarding the role of research units—either independent or inside government—what institutional characteristics and activities help foster research impact on policy? Second, what practical advice can be provided on what could work most effectively in different contexts?
c. Links: How do different types of network and policy research communities influence policy-making in developing countries? Do different sorts of policy networks, work better in different environments? Do legitimacy and trust make a difference, and how can they be strengthened?
d. External influences: The cases illustrated a number of innovative ways to ensure research has a greater policy impact. Future research might address the impact of local and international politics and processes, as well as the impact of general donor policies and specific research-funding instruments.

Answers to some of these questions would provide practical advice to researchers and research institutes on what could work in different contexts.

Endnotes

1. Hart, J. The Inverse Care Law. *Lancet*, 1971, 1:405-12.
2. Julius Court and John Young. The RAPID Framework for Assessing Research-Policy Links. London, Overseas Development Institute, 2002 (available at: http://www.odi.org.uk/RAPID/Events/DSA_BRP_2004/Docs/RAPID_Framework.pdf, accessed 24 June 2008).
3. Meessen B, *et al*. Concept paper on the 4K framework. Unpublished paper. Belgium, Institute of Tropical Medicine, Antwerp, 2007.
4. Lavis, J. *et al*. Assessing country-level efforts to link research to action. *Bulletin of the World Health Organization*, August 2006, 84 8..
5. Scott, V. *et al*. Research to action to address inequities: the experience of the Cape Town Equity Gauge, *International Journal for Equity in Health*, 2008, 7:6 doi:10.1186/1475-9276-7-6.
6. Court and Young 2002. Op. cit.
7. See, for example, David Evans. Hierarchy of evidence: a framework for ranking evidence evaluating health care interventions. *South Australia Journal of Clinical Nursing*, 2003, 12: 77–84.
8. Another example can be found at http://www.shef.ac.uk/scharr/ir/units/systrev/hierarchy.htm (accessed 24 June 2008).
9. Lavis *et al. Op. cit.*

Annex

Methodology for case study writing [1]

1. Steps to an evidence-based case study

These points are intended to provide an overall guidance to case study design. Not all may be applicable to the case study to be captured. The case study is not supposed to replace technical or scientific documentation, rather to complement it by describing the gathering and the use of evidence in a narrative, anecdotal form. The level of technical detail should be varied based upon the intended audience for the case study.

The actual writing of the case study should keep in mind the following points:

- It should have a clear and precise title.
- Tell it like a story and develop the story in user friendly text.
- It is important to keep the key messages up front and start with a summary and conclusion.
- The total summary should be no more than 200 to 300 words.
- Think about the case study as presenting a meal in a restaurant: both the information content and the presentation should stimulate customers to consume.
- The total case study should be 4 - 6,000 words (approx. 8-12 A4 pages).
- Be explicit and precise both about the 'question or problem' and the 'purpose'.
- Address your target audience—in this case, high-level policy-makers from ministries of health, and national and international partners from academia and the nongovernmental sector engaged in undertaking and applying policy-relevant health research with a focus on equity.
- How is a case study different from any other article or technical review? The case study is about 'convincing' your audience about the impact of an intervention or an idea; case study writing allows more 'flexibility' than a standard technical review in the presentation of the evidence; even though the case study should be evidence-based, the focus of the case study can be on the story being told and not on the evidence which can be presented only as background material. The case study is about presenting 'arguments' for 'persuasion'; it is an 'anticipatory marketing' tool. The case study is about the methodology and process as well as about the story-line.
- End by highlighting those lessons that are generalizable and can be transferred to another setting.

2. Template for a case study

Title
The title should be clear and precise enough to capture the story-line.

Summary
The total length of an executive summary should be 200 to 300 words and include key messages and conclusions.

Question (problem) definition
Define the exact question that is to be addressed precisely and explicitly. If the problem is related to health

---

1   Adapted from: Handbook for evidence-based working and case study writing. WHO, Regional Office for Europe, 2005 (pages 65-70). Available at: http://www.euro.who.int/document/ENI/Handbook_case_study.pdf

equity, define the concept of equity[2] used in this context, and what methods and indicators are used to measure equity/inequity. Define if a 'proactive' or 'reactive' approach is used.

The section on problem definition should be used if the case study is being written to address a specific 'problem' (as opposed to writing a case study to address a pre-determined purpose or a set of aims).

Purpose (aims)
Define the exact question that is to be addressed precisely and explicitly. This section should be used if the case study is being written to address a pre-determined purpose (as opposed to addressing a problem). State if the purpose of the text is for understanding, convincing, or demonstrating.

Assumptions
State explicitly if the case study write-up is based upon a set of assumptions. These assumptions will colour the perspectives of the audience in their perception of the case study.

Introduction and brief history
Provide a programme/project/intervention description, context, history of birth, and justification.

Background and context
It is important to describe the context up front in the case study. The description of the strategy for gathering, analysing and using evidence should reflect the context described in this section. The description of the context can make it clear, if the evidence is context specific or whether it is generalizable or transferable. This section should be used to highlight potential conflicts with other existing programmes, interventions or desired outcomes.

Prevailing political climate and agenda setting

Set the scene and examine the social and political influences and trends current at the time of programme inception and implementation, using items from the checklist below, as relevant.
- The history of emergence of a problem
- The political and social climate
- Political commitment to the goal of improving health equity
- Whether a bottom up or top down programme
- Time frame
- Demographic patterns in the region
- Economic situation in the region
- Dominant political agendas
- NGO influences, if any
- Public opinion/debate

---

2   There are several definitions of equity. We include two examples:
   - Equity: Principle of being fair to all, with reference to a defined and recognized set of values. Equity in health implies that ideally everyone should have a fair opportunity attain their full health potential and more pragmatically, that no one should be disadvantaged from achieving this potential, i.e. everyone should have geographical and financial access to available resources in health care.
     Source: Glossary of the European Observatory on Health Systems and Policies, URL: http://www.euro.who.int/observatory/Glossary/ (May 2007).
   - Equity is the absence of avoidable or remediable differences among groups of people, whether those groups are defined socially, economically, demographically, or geographically. Health inequities therefore involve more than inequality with respect to health determinants, access to the resources needed to improve and maintain health or health outcomes. They also entail a failure to avoid or overcome inequalities that infringe on fairness and human rights norms.
     Source: http://www.who.int/healthsystems/topics/equity/en/ (May 2007)

Look at the influences and events that helped turn a social problem into a political challenge, using items from the checklist below, as relevant
- Who were the major advocate groups?
- Alliances between lobbying groups
- How did the advocacy process take place?
- What were the catalysts for public debate?
- What did public debate focus on?
- How did improving health equity become a policy goal?
- Response to the public debate from the Government, NGOs, business, consumers?
- Major opportunities seen during this process
- Primary obstacles and barriers encountered
- Lessons learned

The sections on background and context should total a maximum of 300–600 words, or 1–2 A4 pages.

Development of strategy and development of evidence

This section elaborates on the methods used to gather, analyse and use evidence as well as how the evidence was graded. Since the context has been described and presented in an earlier section, present the evidence in a context-sensitive manner. Define transparently the sources of information used to build arguments. The total length of this section should be about 400 words or 1 A4 page.

- Data and evidence enable analysis of equity aspects, such as disaggregation of data or information by various relevant social stratifiers or indicators of social exclusion, such as sex, socio-economic status, age, geographical location (rural/urban), ethnicity, employment status?
- Is evidence available at political, programme and/or community level?
- Is the evidence generalizable and transferable (from one Member State to another/ within one Member State)?
- Should there be a different approach for different countries?
- What is classified as good evidence?

Implementation and use (policy formulation and/or amendment)

How was the existing policy amended or implemented? Use items from the checklist below, as relevant.
- The ultimate event that provoked a policy response
- How did policy proposal originate and what were the main goals?
- Collaboration and funding
- Recruitment and training
- The process of policy formulation or amendment (what evidence base was used?)
- Roles played by health ministers, community and consumer groups, private sector
- Impact of the public debate
- What role did the local health authority play (initiator/supporter/opponent)?
- Components of the policy research, education, services
- Policy announcement — political timing?
- Programme advertisement and promotion
- Partnerships and alliances

What health outcomes were achieved?

- Have the intended outcomes of the programme/project/intervention been achieved? Also describe the magnitude of changes.
- Have the expected outcomes related to equity been achieved?
- What outcome indicators were used?
- What indicators were used to assess equity?

Look at what was actually achieved as a result of the public policy experience
- Was evaluation built into the implementation process? Monitoring, especially of health equity, on a continuous basis?
- Did health concerns become stronger due to this policy change?
- Did structures/institutions change?
- Did the overall resource patterns change?
- Did public opinion change?
- Has the next attempt to influence policy been made easier?
- How were staff de-briefed and the lessons transmitted?
- Why would you call this policy/programme/intervention a success?

Capture 'better' practices (generalizability)

Having described the context and the evidence gathering, it is now important to analyse how context specific the outcomes are. It is important to highlight those results which are transferable or at least separate those elements which are generalizable.

Challenges and lessons learned

Outline the major barriers and challenges faced and generalize, if possible, the lessons learned in order to capture better practices for future reference. Describe specific measures taken to overcome the barriers.
- Barriers and failed efforts, especially to improving health equity
- Funding
- Training/volunteers
- How to be sustainable?
- Limitations of technology
- Gathering of information and/or evidence
- Transferability of evidence

Evaluate programme effectiveness

Prepare this as the evidence base to guide future decision-making and policy efforts.

Conclusions and final results

Assuming that the strategy is now accepted, explain how it was implemented:
- What changes were made in administration to implement policy?
- Were other programmes eliminated/downgraded to allow for this policy?
- Were new funds allocated?
- How long did it take to implement the policy?
- Was the 'spirit' of the policy observed?

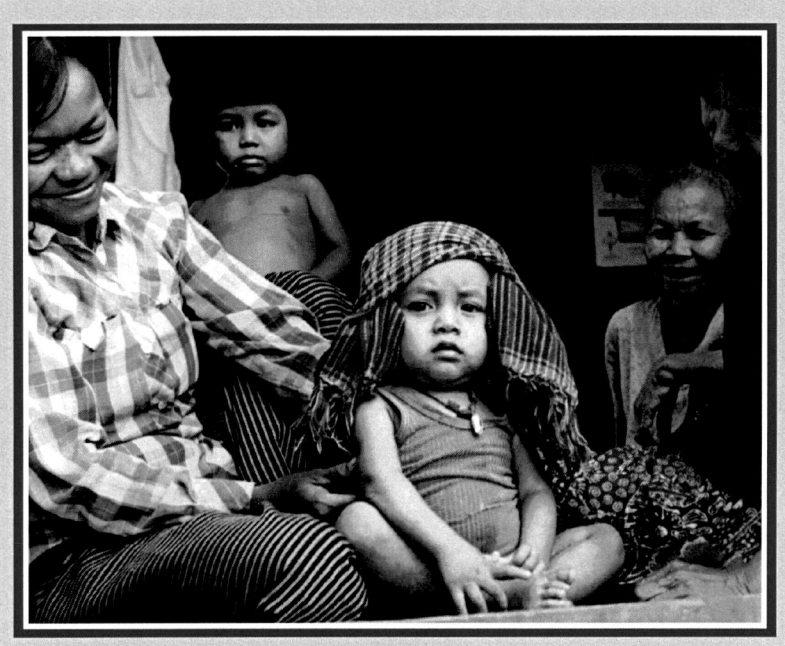

Health financing strategies to improve access to health services for the poor in Cambodia: from pilot to policy and action—A case study of Health Equity Funds

Por Ir[1], Maryam Bigdeli[2]

1. Summary

Health inequities exist worldwide. Addressing them requires more evidence-informed policy-making. But reliable evidence is scarce and often not used by policy-makers. Health equity is an essential objective of health sector reforms, and health financing is one of its most important components.

In this study, we examine health financing strategies designed to improve access to health services for Cambodia's poor, in particular Health Equity Funds (HEFs) and draw lessons on using evidence to develop policies that promote equity. We use a '4K' framework to describe the HEF policy development process in Cambodia and illustrate how a pilot project can become part of national health policy.

Cambodian health policy clearly stipulates a commitment to ensuring equitable access to quality health care for all citizens, especially the poor. Health sector development in Cambodia is now geared towards improving equity in access to and utilization of quality services. The failure of efforts to make public health services free for all urged the Ministry of Health to look for alternative financing strategies. Therefore, several health financing mechanisms for improving access to health services, particularly for the poor, have been developed and implemented. These include user fees and exemptions, contracting, health equity funds and community-based health insurance.

User fees improved the performance of public health facilities but became a barrier for the poor to access public health services, especially at the secondary and tertiary levels, because the exemption policy failed. Contracting boosted the use of health services by improving quality and management, but the increase in use highlighted the problem of access for the poor. In this context, HEFs were piloted as a purchaser-to-pay model for hospital fees and other access-related costs (K1). Evidence of the success of HEF pilots was generated by evaluations and case studies (K2) and widely disseminated (K3). Progressively, HEFs have been replicated in many places and have become part of Cambodia's national health financing policy (K4).

The concept of HEFs is widely accepted and supported, at least for the short and medium-term, by all actors. Many donors are willing to allocate more funds. Government budget is also

---

1 Institute of Tropical Medicine Antwerp, Belgium
2 World Health Organization, Cambodia

identified and allocated. However, a full HEF policy is still lacking. Such a policy could ensure effective scaling up of HEFs. More research is needed to further shape HEF policy, as well as overall health financing policy, and to achieve health equity goals.

The uptake of HEF by the Cambodian health policy was determined by three important and synergistic factors: a conducive political context; credibility and timeliness of HEF evidence; and commitment and good relationship among actors.

2. Introduction

Health systems in many countries continue to be inequitable. They provide more and higher quality services to the rich, who need them less, than to the poor, who often fail to get them. To address health inequities, a joint effort must be made to ensure that health systems more effectively reach disadvantaged groups or the poor. It requires evidence-informed policy-making to improve health and reduce health inequalities, particularly in low and middle income countries.

Recent international policy debates pose health equity as an objective of health sector reforms, yet targets to improve averages mask increasing divergence between the outcomes of the rich and the poor. Health financing is a key component of health sector reform that can effectively address health inequities. Reliable evidence on efficient and equitable health financing in different settings, however, is sparse.

Cambodia has been the testing ground for multiple health financing innovations to improve access for the population to public health services, especially the poor. The development of HEFs is an innovation to promote health equity and reduce poverty. Supported by evidence, these funds have progressed from a few pilots to become part of Cambodia's national health financing policy.

This case study presents health financing strategies to improve access to health services for the poor in Cambodia, focusing on HEFs. We describe the HEF policy development process to illustrate how a pilot project became part of national health policy, and draw lessons on how evidence can be used to inform policies and actions that promote health equity.

2.1 Concepts and methods

In the literature, the term "evidence" often refers to research-related or empirical evidence. In this study, we use a definition that confers broader meaning to "evidence", to include research, knowledge and information, ideas and interests, and finally, politics and economics.

Policy can be defined as a broad statement of goals, objectives and means that create a framework for actions. Health policy is a network of interrelated decisions which together form an approach or strategy in relation to practical issues concerning health services delivery.

The theory of evidence-based policy is growing. Policy-making is not linear or rarely an event or an explicit set of decisions. Rather it tends to evolve through an interactive process and involve a wide range of actors. Several frameworks for analysis of research-policy links have been proposed. Most of these identify three common factors that determine the influence of evidence on policy: (1) the content of evidence; (2) the political context of the policy and evidence; and (3) actors and the interaction between them.

In this study, we use a framework that considers knowledge as evidence to analyse the process of HEF-related policy development in Cambodia. This '4K framework' describes four stages, each of which is analysed by the determining factors of content, context, and actors. These stages comprise K1: exploiting existing knowledge; K2: creating new knowledge or innovations; K3: disseminating the new knowledge (evidence brokering); K4: adopting and using the new knowledge.

We analysed all available HEF-related documents to gather existing evidence and policy related to HEF to construct the story of HEF development. In addition, we interviewed 20 key informants using a semi-structured questionnaire to learn about their involvement in the HEF policy process, their knowledge on HEF-related evidence, and their interest, position and influence on HEF policy. The informants include policy-makers from the Ministries of Health, Economy and Finance, and Planning, as well as representatives from donor agencies, international non-governmental organisations (NGOs), and consultants and researchers, all of whom have been involved in HEF policy development. Information from document analysis, key informant interviews, and the knowledge of the research team were carefully compared with the help of a review team with members from the Ministry of Health, the National Institute of Public Health and WHO.

3. Background

3.1 Equity and Cambodian health policy

Health sector development in Cambodia is strongly geared towards improving equity in access to and utilization of quality services, especially for the poor, and protecting them against the impoverishing effects of ill health. Reflecting article 72 of the National Constitution, the Mission of the Cambodian Ministry of Health calls for "commitment to ensure sector-wide equitable quality health care for all the people of Cambodia through targeting resources especially to the poor and to areas of greatest need."

The Ministry of Health's National Health Strategic Plan 2003-2007 (HSSP) embraces several pro-poor health financing strategies, one of which is to allocate financial resources to improve the accessibility of health services for the poor through alternative health financing schemes.

The National Poverty Reduction Strategy 2003-2005 (NPRS) emphasizes the need for targeting public resources to the poor in the health sector to promote health equity. It highlights three key strategies aiming to reduce financial barriers of access for the poor, as well as improve management capacity within the health sector. These include:

1. regulatory mechanisms for prices through official user fee schemes with community participation in setting prices, identifying the poor for exemptions and monitoring quality;

2. development and implementation of HEFs to further promote access to priority services and protect the poor against catastrophic health expenditure; and
3. contracting with NGOs to deliver basic health services in poor and remote areas.

The National Strategic Development Plan 2006-2010 (NSDP) considers HEFs a key health sector strategy to promote equity and reduce poverty. It calls for further expansion and strengthening of HEFs to help the poor access public health services, and further exploration to find sustainable ways to help the poor.

3.2 The evolution of health financing in Cambodia

In the framework of health sector reform, health financing reform in Cambodia has a rich history in which several key strategies have been developed and implemented (Figure 1). Key features of each scheme and their impacts on equity are summarised in Table 1.

Figure 1: Development of Different Health Financing Schemes in Cambodia

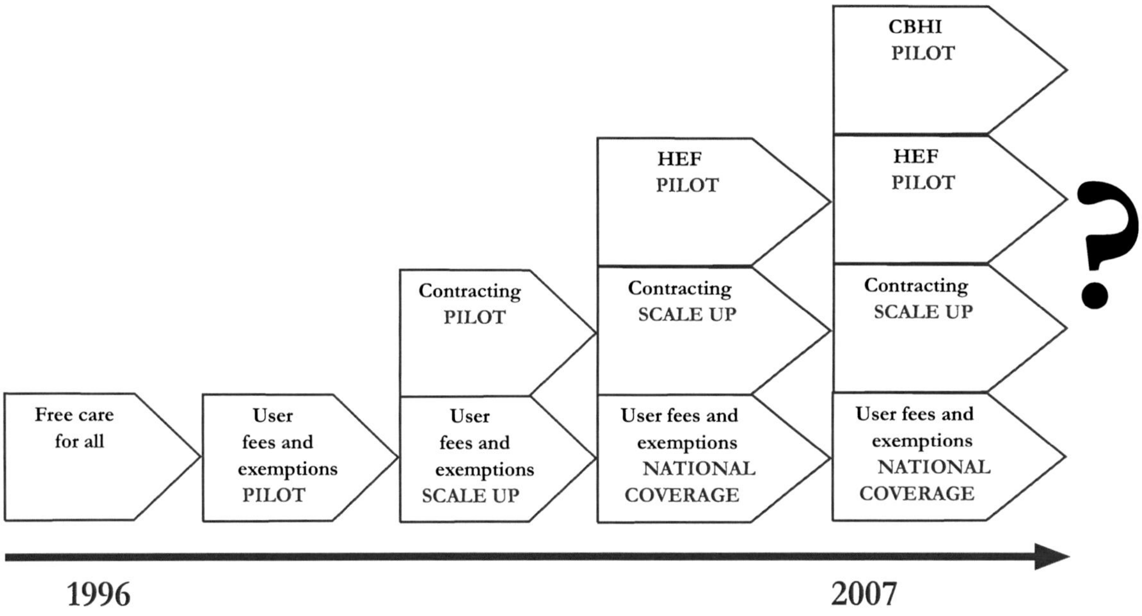

3.3 Free care for all

From 1980 to 1989, after decades of civil war and the devastation of the country by the Khmer Rouge, the Cambodian Ministry of Health started reconstructing and rehabilitating the public health system. A strengthening and development period from 1989 to 1995 saw substantial investments by the Government and development partners, as well as growth in the private sector. Services in public facilities were free of charge, but informal payments were common. The services offered by government facilities were of poor quality and often not accessible by many people. This resulted in low utilisation of public health facilities, to the benefit of the largely unregulated private sector. Health care expenditure was consequently high, mainly paid out-of-pocket, and caused many households to go into debt or lose productive assets.

Various surveys confirmed the low utilisation of public facilities and showed high health care costs and burden for the households (Box 1).

Box 1: Summary of findings

Health Care Demand Survey 1996:
- 57% of patients opted for self-medication through the purchase of drugs from pharmacies or private practitioners who were mostly unlicensed and untrained.
- Expenditure on health care constituted 22% of total household expenditure, and those in the lowest income quintile paid a higher percentage (28%) of income on health care.
- About half of patients borrowed money to pay for health care costs.

Cambodian Socio-Economic Survey 1997:
- 27% of ill Cambodians did not seek medical help or were self-medicated.
- Only 24% of patients sought care from a public provider, but almost a third visited private providers.
- There was high out-of-pocket health care expenditure even in public facilities that were supposedly free of charge: one outpatient visit to a commune clinic or district health centre took a third of annual non-food spending for someone in the poorest quintile, and an inpatient visit to a public hospital cost more than twice their annual non-food spending.
- Household expenditure on health care was estimated at 11% of total household expenditure.

Health and Landlessness Mini-Study 2000:
- For the first treatment, 66% used private sector services and 30% used public services. 74% borrowed money to pay for health care.
- Household health expenditure was the major cause of landlessness in Cambodia.

Sources: National Public Health and Research Institute, 1998; World Bank, 1999; OXFAM, 2000.

To respond to the situation, the Ministry of Health explored alternative financing strategies. The adoption of the National Charter on Health Financing in 1996 was a policy breakthrough, providing a legal framework for implementing different health financing schemes.

3.4 User fees and exemption

Formal user fees were piloted in several government health facilities in 1997. The aim was to generate extra revenues and facilitate good management to improve quality of services and reduce unofficial payments. Safeguards to prevent negative effects of user fees on access for the poor were introduced alongside user fee schemes. These included an exemption policy, community participation in setting prices and identifying the poor for exemptions, and full fee schedules posted at the entrance of each facility.

To date almost all public health facilities have implemented user fees, with varying results. Studies showed that user fees brought some benefits in developing management controls and generating revenues to improve the performance of government health facilities, but they became a barrier for the poor to access public services, especially hospital services. Exemption at health centres worked relatively well, but failed to protect the poor at hospitals. The exemption rates at the government hospitals were very low and mainly benefited wealthier Cambodians. The Cambodian Socio-Economic Survey 1997 showed only 12.2% of the poorest quintile obtained free treatment from government health facilities while 26.2% of the richest quintile paid no fees.

The failure of the exemption policy was due to the conflict between a viable exemption scheme and a viable salary incentive scheme, as 49% of income from user fees was earmarked for staff incentives. Exempting a poor patient meant a financial loss for staff. The lack of clear procedures and tools for exemptions was also considered a reason for the failure of the policy.

3.5 Contracting

To address the issue of low quality and low utilisation of public health services, contracting arrangements were developed as a supply-side financing strategy. Several contracting models were tested with the objective of improving the performance of public health facilities.

In 1999 the Ministry of Health piloted the contracting of health services delivery to NGOs in five remote districts, with funding provided through an Asian Development Bank loan project. Two operational research models of contracting were tested: two 'contracting-out'[3] districts and three 'contracting-in'[4] districts, with four control districts. The evaluation showed that both models outperformed the existing system in terms of increased utilisation by the poor and reduced household expenditure on health care. The contracting was relatively expensive, however, and outsourcing management to NGOs was thought to undermine institutional development and put the sustainability of the model at risk. Balancing those constraints and the effectiveness of the model, the Ministry of Health used a modified design to extend contracting to 11 poor and remote districts in the second phase (2003-2007).

Other contracting arrangements were also being tested. These included efforts in Takeo provincial hospital in 1997 by the Swiss Red Cross; the New Deal in Thmar Pouk and Sotnikum districts by Médecins sans Frontières (MSF) and UNICEF; and a similar contracting scheme in eight health districts (including Sotnikum) in 2004 by Belgian Technical Cooperation. In these arrangements incentives were provided based on performance and output indicators, but they relied on the existing government management structure. The performance of the contracted facilities improved sharply and informal fees were no longer charged, but the issue of equity of access for the poor was again raised.

3.6 Health Equity Funds

Health Equity Funds are a demand-side financing mechanism used to promote access to priority public health services for the poor in an environment where user fees are charged. HEF beneficiaries are identified according to eligibility criteria, either at the community level, before health care demands are made (pre-identification)[5] or at the health facilities themselves,

---

3   NGO contractors were given complete responsibility including hiring and firing staff, setting wages, procuring and distributing drugs and supplies and organizing and staffing facilities.
4   NGO contractors worked within the government health system to strengthen it, but without hiring/firing power.
5   For pre-identification, eligible poor households were systematically assessed at their home based on observable proxy means tests prior to the episode of illness.

through interviews (post-identification)[6]. At the health facility, the eligible poor patients get full or partial support from HEF for the cost of user fees[7], transport cost and other costs during hospitalisation.

HEF pilots were initiated in 2000. They were found to be effective in improving equity in access to health services and potentially protecting the poor from high health care costs. HEFs were also considered an efficient way to transfer resources to the poor since they purchased the already heavily subsidized public services, yet incurred lower-than-average per-patient hospital bills. These convincing results drew a lot of attention from NGOs, international agencies, donors and policy-makers. HEFs were replicated in other places and produced similar results.

In 2003, HEFs became an integral component of Cambodia's Health Sector Support Programme and National Poverty Reduction Strategy. The Ministry of Health developed its Strategic Framework for Equity Funds, laying out principles for design, management, and evaluation of HEFs. To translate the strategic framework into a concrete policy implementation tool, the Ministry of Health also developed a National Equity Fund Implementation and Monitoring Framework.

In late 2006 the Ministry of Health and Ministry of Economy and Finance jointly issued a *Prakas* (directive) stipulating the allocation of State budget to subsidize the poor in accessing public health services through reimbursement of user fees. The Ministry of Health immediately set up exemption reimbursement schemes in six national hospitals and eight health districts, which are also called Health Equity Funds. To date 42 hospital-based and several health centre-based HEF schemes[8] have been implemented.

3.7 Health Insurance

Along with the above health financing innovations, community-based health insurance (CBHI) has also been tested in Cambodia since 1999 by Groupe de Recherche et d'Echanges Technologiques (GRET), an international NGO. The result of the pilot was not persuasive enough to attract policy-makers' attention; even with the modest annual premium of US$ 1.5 per person, GRET could only enrol 167 families (711 persons) in their CBHI scheme in more than 1 year. More recently, other initiatives by GRET and other NGOs were more successful and point the way to a social health insurance health policy element.

A master plan for social health insurance provides broad guidelines and strategies to move towards social health insurance. A committee of key stakeholders was formed to advocate the development of social health insurance initiatives with universal coverage through compulsory health insurance in a social security framework for public and private sector salaried workers and their dependents; voluntary insurance through CBHI schemes for informal sector workers; and social assistance through HEFs for non-economically active and indigent populations. A national guideline for CBHI has been developed.

---

6   Post-identification takes place in the hospital premises, when patients ask for it or when they are referred for financial assistance.
7   Many HEFs reimburse only hospital fees while some cover health centre services.
8   This includes 14 hospitals with only Exemption Reimbursement funded by the state budget.

Table 1: Summary of key features of the four health financing schemes and their impact on equity

	User Fees and Exemption	Contracting	Health Equity Funding	Community-based Health Insurance
Key objective	Generate extra revenues for public health facilities to improve services.	Improve the performance of public health facilities.	Improve access to health services for the poor.	Prevent catastrophic health expenditure.
Rationale	Under-funding of public health facilities; stop unofficial payments.	Low quality and low utilisation of public services; outsourcing services to NGOs.	User fees become a barrier for access for the poor; exemption policy fails to protect the poor.	Social health protection; financial sustainability.
Coverage (As of September 2007)	Almost all health facilities.	11 remote health districts with ADB loan and 9 with Belgian grant (~25%).	42 hospital-based and several HC-based schemes (27 with external fund, 14 by government budget (~50%).	6 health district-based schemes.
Expected impact on equity	Through (unfunded) exemptions for the poor at facilities.	Indirectly through improved service delivery in remote and underserved areas.	By providing financial access to health services for the poor.	Indirectly through preventing impoverishment for members in rural areas.
Local evidence of impact on equity	Improved equitable access at health centres.	Higher utilisation and lower household expenditure for low socio-economic group.	Improved access to hospital care for the poor and mitigation of health care burden.	Still to be assessed.

4. From pilot to policy: the case of health equity funding

4.1 K1-exploiting existing knowledge: birth of HEF idea

In developing countries, knowledge is often sourced from international experiences and applied with or without adaptation to the local context. HEF in Cambodia was locally generated to address a national problem.

In late 1999, the Urban Health Project was created to improve access to basic health services for the urban poor in Phnom Penh. Two health rooms were set up to provide primary curative consultations and to some preventive care, and to refer severe and complicated cases to nearby government hospitals. Some clients who needed to be referred, however, could not afford to pay the costs and abstained from treatment, or fell into debt. An Equity Fund was therefore created in August 2000 to pay for the costs of referral services, including the reimbursement of 70% of user fees, as well as transport and food costs.

Similarly, the New Deal in Sotnikum and Thmar Pouk health districts were launched respectively in late 1999 and early 2000. Initiated and funded by Médecins sans Frontières and UNICEF in collaboration with the Ministry of Health, it attempted to break the vicious cycle of underpaid health staff and poor quality, underutilised public health services. The higher user fees that were introduced became barriers to access for the poor, particularly for hospitalization. A special fund was created and entrusted to a local NGO to identify the eligible poor patients and to partially or fully pay the hospital user fees and related costs on their behalf. These pilots were called *Mulnithi Sangkrus Chun Krey Krar* (a fund to save the poor). Later the name 'Health Equity Fund' was applied.

4.2 K2-Creating new knowledge or innovation: results from HEF pilots

As described, evaluations and studies of the pilots showed persuasive evidence in terms of promoting access to hospital services for the poor and their potential effect on protecting the poor from impact of health care cost.

4.2.1 Evidence from the first HEF pilots

The first year evaluation report of the Urban Health Project concluded that a HEF could effectively help many poor patients overcome financial barriers to access hospital services and get treated early rather than risk a worsening of the condition. By doing so, it protected the poor against the high costs of health care and prevented them from selling assets or taking out loans to pay health costs. However, the limited benefit package provided by the HEF undermined its effectiveness. The incomplete reimbursement (70%) of the referral cost and limited welfare support (transport, food) still caused an access barrier for many poor Cambodians. Furthermore, the partial reimbursement made some providers unwilling to accept HEF beneficiaries or, if accepted, they treated them for only what they paid for. The evaluation also recommended that the HEF be managed by a local NGO to minimise temptations for financial mismanagement and favouritism.

The early results of HEFs in Thmar Pouk and Sotnikum showed that HEFs managed by a third party NGO can effectively improve financial access to hospital services for the poor and consequently promote utilization of public health services. Patients supported by HEFs were genuinely poor and their numbers increased over time, without reducing use by fee-paying patients. It also showed that HEFs were a cost-effective strategy to transfer resources to the poor. Despite these positive effects, many poor patients did not reach the hospital because of other barriers to access, mainly lack of awareness of HEFs or uncertainty of their entitlements. The post-identification arrangement was seen as the main problem, which negated the benefits of bringing poor patients straight to the hospital (which would entail fewer delays in seeking care and reduce the wasting of money in the private sector or the use of other risky coping strategies).

Based on the Thmar Pouk and Sotnikum experiences, the following requisites for replication of HEFs were laid down:

- User fees for poor patients, if charged, should be financed from a fund that is created for

this purpose (a HEF), so that health staff gets the same income from treating poor and non-poor patients;
- The health facility where the HEF is implemented must be credible and well functioning in the eyes of the population and able to provide basic quality health care;
- Apart from user fees, other access costs should be paid for from the HEF, in particular transport cost and food expenses;
- The HEF should be managed by a transparent and committed body that has the capacity to identify and support the poorest patients, and is not vulnerable to favouritism.

4.2.2 Accumulated evidence from other HEF pilots

The HEF model was soon replicated in other places with some design modifications. These new pilots reinforced the emerging evidence on the effectiveness of HEFs, and indicated that similar results can be obtained with different designs of HEF. Finally, they documented new findings on administrative arrangements, pre-identification and access to tertiary care.

Box 2: Summary of accumulated evidence from new HEF pilots

- Village-based pre-identification is feasible and cost-effective.
- Pre-identification seems to be superior to post-identification in promoting use by the poor through increased awareness about HEFs and greater certainty regarding their entitlements. However pre-identification is not viable on its own. Post-identification remains necessary as a complement to pre-identification.
- Limited benefit packages may undermine the effectiveness of HEFs. In addition to support for secondary level care, the cost of tertiary care referrals should be included in the benefit package.
- A mixed committee composed of representatives from the community, pagodas, local health authority and NGOs taking charge (or at least monitoring and evaluating) of the HEF is both effective and inexpensive.
- The management arrangement of the Provincial Health Department in charge of the fund and an NGO for identifying the poor worked well.
- Participation by the local community in design, implementation, monitoring and evaluation not only greatly reduced the administrative cost but also enhanced local ownership of the HEF, which in turn increased the likelihood of sustainability.

4.3 K3-Brokering new knowledge: dissemination of evidence from HEF pilots

Brokering knowledge is a strategy to close the gap between evidence, policy and action. It promotes the uptake of evidence for policy formulation and implementation. Knowledge brokering is a two-way process that aims to encourage policy-makers to be more responsive to research findings and stimulate researchers to conduct policy-relevant research and translate their findings to be meaningful to policy-makers.

In Cambodia, evidence is transferred to policy-makers through a wider network under the framework of sector-wide management (Figure 2). The monthly meetings of the Technical Working Group-Health (TWG-H) at the central level or the Provincial Technical Working Group-Health at the provincial level allow the Ministry of Health and its partners to discuss and share information. MEDICAM, an association of NGOs active in health, provides a forum for their members to meet, discuss and share information, and represents the NGOs in the TWG-H.

Additionally, there are many sub-working groups or committees or task forces that were created to gather evidence to develop specific guidelines or policies. These groups report to theTWG-H. *Ad hoc* meetings, workshops and conferences are frequent in Cambodia, and study tours to observe results in the field are also often used as practical and direct ways of informing policy-makers.

Figure 2: Evidence-policy communication network in health care in Cambodia

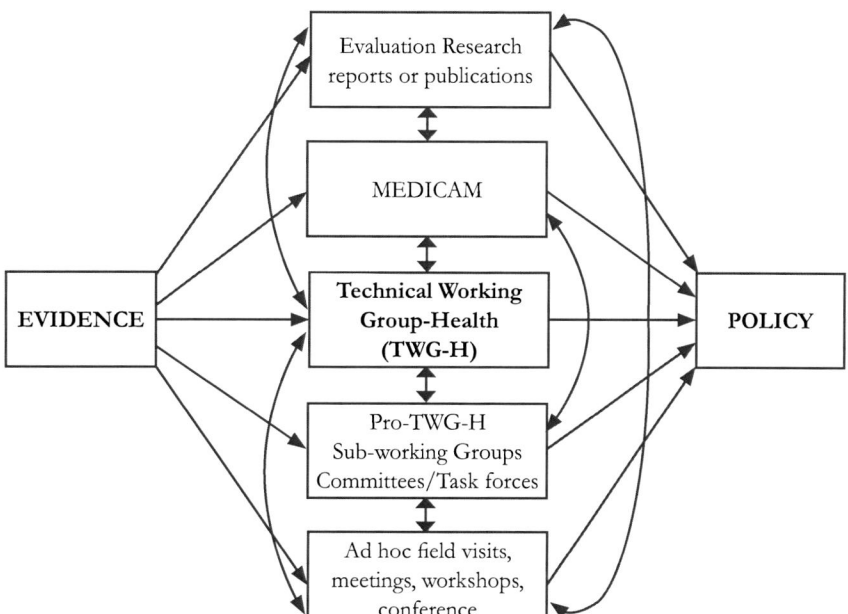

One of the strategies of the Sotnikum New Deal was to involve as many key actors as possible in the decision-making process to create a platform for discussions and a broad basis of ownership, which would enhance chances to have an impact of the model on national health policy. To reach these aims, a steering committee that included policy-makers from the Government and the supporting partners was set up. In addition to its regular meetings that allowed members to learn about the model through direct participation and field visits, the steering committee discussed the results of the HEF scheme in two workshops. Publications about the New Deal and HEF results in Sotnikum appeared in local and international publications related to access to health services and health equity.

Dissemination of evidence from the first HEF pilots was crucial to draw the attention of key policy-makers and donors to HEFs and stimulate a policy debate at the national level. MSF, UNICEF and WHO played leading roles at that stage. All the health financing innovations were extensively discussed in the first Joint Annual Performance Review, a venue for the Ministry of Health and its partners to assess progress in health sector and define priorities.

4.4 K4-Adopting and using new knowledge: scaling-up and harmonisation of HEFs

Adoption and use of findings or evidence is a crucial step for research to reach its final outcomes. The stakeholders who first adopted evidence from early pilots of HEF were those who replicated the pilots and tested new models to produce further evidence. Those stakeholders had a direct interest in implementing HEFs to reach social and equity goals. UNICEF's interest was to increase efficiency of their input by shifting its direct financial support to the hospital, in addition to resolving the problem of the low exemption rate. HealthNet International and Enfants et Développement adopted the HEF concept because it answered their question on effective ways to pay user fees for the poor.

Some Cambodian policy-makers were convinced of the benefits of HEFs from the start, but the Ministry of Health formally adopted them at a later stage. The uptake of the experience was explicit in 2002 when the HEF concept was integrated into the Health Sector Reform Project (HSRP) and the Poverty Reduction Strategy Paper (PRSP). That adoption was a breakthrough to promote scaling up of HEF country-wide. In summary, the adoption of the HEF evidence was successful because: (1) HEFs were an effective solution to the failure of exemption; (2) HEFs promoted equity by nature and therefore fitted well with the Ministry of Health's pro-poor policy; and (3) HEFs mobilised additional resources for government health facilities.

There were early debates around HEFs among donor agencies, according to key informants. Opponents argued that HEFs are just charity and not likely to be efficient and sustainable. Only in 2003 was a consensus obtained and donors started to designate funds for HEFs.

To give those donors clear guidance on the future development of HEFs, the Ministry of Health developed the Strategic Framework for Equity Funds and a National Equity Fund Implementation and Monitoring Framework through a thorough consultation process. All HEF stakeholders were consulted and experiences from the HEF pilots were carefully examined and included. The challenge of the policy document was to create an environment in which the older HEFs could continue and newer HEFs could be created under various and sometimes contradictory funding constraints (donors and the State budget, pooled and un-pooled financing arrangements).

To cater to these needs, the final framework includes three Equity Fund management models: Model 1 with an NGO as implementer[9]; Model 2 with the District Health Office as implementer; and Model 3 without an implementer, but with management being the responsibility of the individual hospital. Models 2 and 3 have not been supported by evidence from the HEF pilots and may need further testing.

By April 2006, 24 hospital-based HEF schemes were under implementation in Cambodia, all financed by external funds but designed and implemented differently. Although they share some common characteristics, there is considerable variation among them. Therefore, as a

---

9   Implementer means the agent responsible for overall management of HEF.

follow-up to the publication of the national framework, several initiatives were taken to harmonise the various schemes.

In 2005 the Ministry of Planning organised a national forum on harmonization of identifying poor households for multisectoral purposes. The tools developed are being field tested. Many technical and financial challenges still exist in achieving nation-wide identification of poor households and to convincing stakeholders to use the system.

In early 2006, the Ministry of Health, with donor support, organised the first National Forum on Health Equity Funds, bringing all key stakeholders together to discuss and share experiences. The aim was to obtain consensus on further actions that would harmonise and improve the efficiency of scaling up HEFs and to refine the HEF policy. The forum reached consensus on the impact of HEFs in improving access to public health services for the poor, but the evidence on mitigating the impoverishing effect of illness on the poor was less clear. Furthermore, key policy aspects of HEFs, such as their beneficiary identification methods, organisation and management models, benefit packages, reliable funding sources, and monitoring and evaluation, remained partly unresolved and needing further research.

In late 2006, the Ministries of Health and of Economy and Finance jointly issued a *Prakas* (directive) to allocate State budget to subsidize health care cost for the poor. The *Prakas* is the first regulatory application of the National Framework and applies Models 2 and 3. It stipulates that the State budget will be allocated through the existing government budget disbursement channels to public health facilities. The funds will be used to reimburse the cost of user fees for exempted poor patients, but transport and food costs are not covered. This *Prakas* is an essential step in gaining support of policy-makers beyond the health sector. This regulation demonstrates the commitment of the Ministry of Economy and Finance to allocate funds for the care of the poor. Effective implementation of this model of HEFs remains to be further assessed and carefully documented.

Currently, the Ministry of Health is also identifying a national fund holder for the implementation of a Japanese grant through the Asian Development Bank. This will be an application of the National Framework's Model 1, which will include a third party purchaser and social assistance funds to cover transport and food costs.

Following issuance of the *Prakas*, several new user fee exemption reimbursement schemes have been developed in 14 district, provincial and national hospitals which had no HEFs. This brings the total number of hospital-based HEF schemes to 42 as of September 2007, covering more than 50% of the country. The monitoring and evaluation process will provide further evidence on all three models regardless of sources of funds.

5. Conclusions

The HEF concept is widely accepted and supported by all stakeholders in Cambodia. Many donors have been willing to allocate funds, and budgetary funds have been allocated to subsidize health care cost for the poor. However, the HEF policy remains to be fully developed to provide a clear framework for effective nationwide scaling up of HEFs. More research is needed to further shape HEF policy, as well as overall health financing policy to achieve health equity goals.

The findings from our study confirm that three main factors determine the uptake of evidence into policy: (1) a political context conducive to the creation, dissemination and adoption of evidence, (2) the credibility and timeliness of HEF evidence, and (3) strong commitment and good relationships among actors. The synergy between these three factors was essential to the uptake of the HEF experience in health policy.

5.1 Political context

Many factors made the political context in Cambodia conducive to HEF pilots and brought HEFs higher on the policy agenda, culminating in their inclusion in the national health financing policy:

1. Cambodian health policy has always adopted a pro-poor approach and set equity as a goal.
2. Successive efforts in health sector reforms to achieve this policy goal, in particular in financing reforms, were not entirely satisfactory.
3. There was emerging evidence on widespread poverty, inadequate access to health services by the poor, and impoverishment from health expenditure.
4. There was conclusive evidence that user fees caused a barrier to access for the poor, especially at hospital level, and the exemption policy in most cases failed to protect the poor.
5. The Cambodian Government was and is supportive of innovative interventions that can address the above issues of poverty and access to health services.

5.2 Content of evidence

Evidence on HEFs has been developed over time, through evaluations and case studies of pilot schemes. While some evidence raised methodological concerns, in the main, the conclusions were strong enough to convince policy-makers and donors to adopt the HEF idea. Several reasons can explain the credibility and timeliness of HEF evidence:

1. HEFs are an efficient and pragmatic concept. They serve the dual objective of ensuring access for poor patients while helping the public health facilities to generate income.
2. HEFs came at the time when Cambodians were open to innovative health financing models. They are not only a response to the failure of exemptions, but also an efficient way to transfer donor funds to the poor and to promote equity in donor projects and programmes.
3. HEFs are a locally generated solution, giving a feeling of ownership to Cambodian health leaders, and are easy to understand and adopt.
4. HEFs do not go against the interests of any one actor. All key informants showed their strong support of HEFs at least for the short and medium terms.

5.3 Actors and links

- Many local and international agencies are active in health sector development in Cambodia. They work in a sector-wide management environment under the guidance of the Ministry of Health.
- Several networks and forums have been created to gather all key health stakeholders to discuss and share their experience and ideas.
- HEF pilots were initiated by international organisations, although the Ministry of Health has been supportive and involved from the beginning.
- The role of the Ministry of Health, other line ministries, and donor agencies became more prominent at the stage of scaling up and harmonisation.

Acknowledgements

We would like to thank Professor Wim Van Damme and Mr Bruno Meessen from the Institute of Tropical Medicine in Antwerp, Belgium, for their contribution to the 4K framework and their insightful comments on the first draft of the case study.

We also express our sincere thanks to all the Review Team members, in particular, Dr Lo Veasna Kiry from the Ministry of Health, Dr Saphorn Vonthanak from the National Institute of Public Health, and Dr Benjamin Lane from WHO, for their contribution to the case study.

We are grateful to all the key informants for dedicating their valuable time for the interviews. Our particular thanks to Dr Steve Fabricant, Ms Anjana Bhushan and Dr Reijo Salmela for their comprehensive comments on the case study and editing of the draft report.

References

1. Akashi H. *et al.* User fees at a public hospital in Cambodia: effects on hospital performance and provider attitudes. *Social Science and Medicine*, 2004, 58: 553-564.
2. Barber S., Bonnet F., Bekedam H. Formalizing under-the-table payments to control out-of-pocket hospital expenditures in Cambodia. *Health Policy and Planning*, 2004, 194.: 199-208.
3. Barker C. *The Health Care Policy Process*. Reprinted copy 2000. SAGE Publications, 1996.
4. Bautista M.C.G. *Health financing schemes in Cambodia: Reaching the poor with quality health services*. Phnom Penh, URC/USAID, 2003.
5. Berwick D.M. *Disseminating innovations in health care*. American Medical Association, 2003, 289(15).
6. Bitran R., *et al. Preserving Equity in Health in Cambodia: Health Equity Funds and Prospects for Replication*. Phnom Penh, World Bank, No date.
7. Bowen S. and Zwi A.B. Pathways to "Evidence-Informed" Policy and Practice: A Framework for Action. *PLoS Medicine* 2005, 27.:e166.
8. Buse K., Mays N., Walt G. *Making Health Policy*. First publication by the London School of Hygiene and Tropical Medicine, 2005.
9. Chettra T. *Existing health financing schemes in Cambodia: Lessons learned and perspectives*. Phnom Penh, URC, 2003.
10. Council for Social Development. *National Poverty Reduction Strategy 2003-2005*. Phnom Penh, Royal Government of Cambodia, 2002.

11. Crewe E. and Young J. *Bridging Research and Policy: Context, Evidence and Links*, ODI Working Paper No 173. London, ODI, 2002.
12. Gwatkin D., Bhuiya A., Victora C. Making health systems more equitable. *Lancet,* 2004, 364:1273-80.
13. Hanney S.R. *et al.* The utilisation of health research in policy-making: concepts, examples, and methods of assessment. BMC Health Research Policy and Systems, 2003, 1:2.
14. Hardeman W. *Considering equity in health sector reform, case study of a New Deal in Sotnikum,* Cambodia. [Master of Arts Thesis]. The Hague, Institute of Social Studies, 2001.
15. Hardeman W, *et al.* Access to health care for all? User fees plus a Health Equity Fund in Sotnikum, Cambodia. Health Policy and Planning, 2004 19: 22-32.
16. Ir P. and Hardeman W., *Health Equity Funds: Improving access to health care for the poor – MSF's experience in Cambodia.* Phnom Penh, Médecins sans Frontières, 2003.
17. Jacob B. and Price N. *Improving access for the poorest to public sector health services: insights from Kirivong Operational Health District in Cambodia.* London, Oxford University Press and The London School of Hygiene and Tropical Medicine, 2005.
18. Knowles J. *An economic evaluation of the Health Care for the Poor Component of the Phnom Penh Urban Health Project.* Phnom Penh, 2001.
19. Lavis J.N., *et al.* Use of research to inform public policy-making. *Lancet,* 2004, 364:1615-21.
20. Le Roy P. *Health Insurance Project for Rural Households in Cambodia.* Phnom Penh, GRET, 2000.
21. Meessen B. *Policy entrepreneurship: the 4-K framework.* Unpublished paper. Antwerp, Institute of Tropical Medicine, 2007.
22. Meessen B. *et al. The New Deal in Cambodia: the second year. Confirmed results, confirmed challenges.* Phnom Penh, MSF, 2002.
23. Ministry of Health, Cambodia. *The national charter on health financing in the Kingdom of Cambodia.* Phnom Penh, Royal Government of Cambodia, 1998.
24. Ministry of Health, Cambodia. *Introducing user fees at public sector health facilities in Cambodia. An overview.* Phnom Penh, Royal Government of Cambodia, 2000.
25. Ministry of Health, Cambodia. *Joint Health Sector Review Report.* Phnom Penh, Royal Government of Cambodia, 2001.
26. Ministry of Health, Cambodia. *Health Sector Strategic Plan 2003-2007.* Phnom Penh, Royal Government of Cambodia, 2002.
27. Ministry of Health, Cambodia. *Strategic framework for equity funds: promoting access to priority health services among the poor. Guiding principles for design, management and evaluation.* Phnom Penh, Royal Government of Cambodia, 2003.
28. Ministry of Health, Cambodia. *National equity fund implementation and monitoring framework.* Phnom Penh, Royal Government of Cambodia, 2005.
29. Ministry of Health, Cambodia. *Report Health Equity Fund Forum.* Phnom Penh, Royal Government of Cambodia, 2006.
30. Ministry of Health, Cambodia. SRC, WHO. *Takeo Provincial Hospital: Pioneering a health financing scheme. Takeo province, Kingdom of Cambodia.* Phnom Penh, Royal Government of Cambodia, 2002.
31. National Public Health and Research Institute, WHO, GTZ. *Health Care Demand Survey.* Phnom Penh, National Public Health and Research Institute, 1998.
32. Nguyen A. *The Svay Rieng Health Equity Fund: A project evaluation.* UNICEF Phnom Penh, and University of Texas School of Public Health, Dallas, 2004.
33. Oxfam. *Health and Landlessness, mini case study.* Oxfam GB Cambodia land study project. Phnom Penh, Oxfam, 2000.
34. Palmer N. *et al.* Health financing to promote access in low income settings–how much do we know? Lancet, 2004, 364:1365-70
35. Royal Government of Cambodia. *National Strategic Development Plan 206-2010.* Phnom Penh, Royal Government of Cambodia, 2006.
36. Van Damme W. and Meessen B.*Sotnikum New Deal, the first year.* Phnom Penh, MSF,2001.

37. Van Kammen J., de Savigny D., Sewankambo N. Using knowledge brokering to promote evidence-based policy-making: the need for support structure. *Bulletin of the World Health Organization*; 2006 848..
38. Wilkinson D., Hollowat J., Fallavier P. *The impact of user fees on access, equity and health provider practices in Cambodia*. Phnom Penh, Ministry of Health, 2001.
39. World Bank. *Cambodia Poverty Assessment*. Phnom Penh, World Bank, 1999.
40. World Health Organization. *Health Equity Fund in Pursat provincial hospital. 6-month evaluation report*. Unpublished draft. Phnom Penh, WHO, 2003.

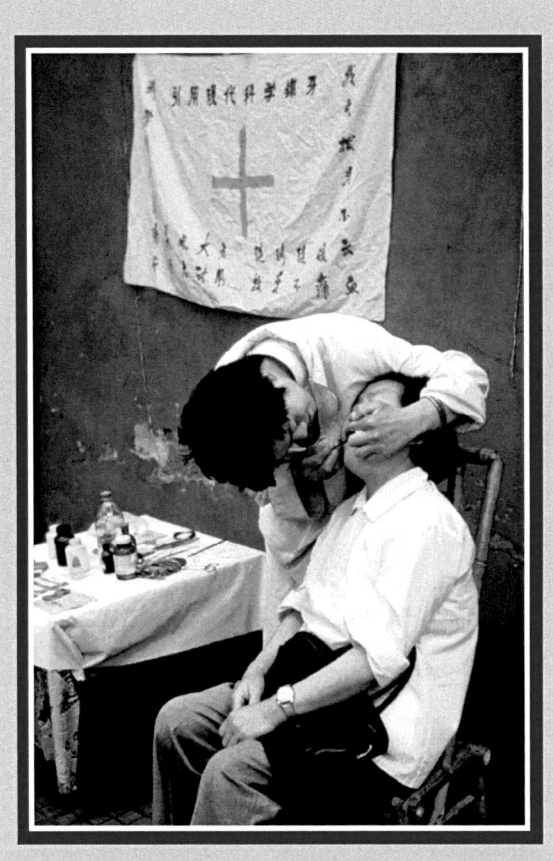

Research, intervention design and policy implementation of the New Rural Cooperative Medical Scheme in Shandong, China

Wang Yan [1], Meng Qingyue [2], Yu Baorong [2], Han Dong [1], Tang Shenglan [3]

1. Background

The purpose of this case study is to report experiences in policy development and implementation for China's largest rural health insurance scheme. Responding to a need to improve the New Rural Cooperative Medical Scheme (NCMS) and especially the health insurance component, researchers and other stakeholders carried out a baseline situation analysis and designed and tested a variety of interventions. The evaluated interventions have guided several important policy changes.

As is well known, the Chinese economy has developed rapidly over the past two and half decades. This rapid economic growth has led to a better quality of life for the Chinese population. Although the overall economic situation has been improved over the past years for both rural and urban areas, gaps in social and economic status between regions and population groups have widened. In 1990, the urban per capita income was 2.2 times higher than the rural per capita income. The difference had increased to 3.2 times by 2003.[1] In general, the eastern industrialized provinces have grown rich, while the central and western provinces remain poor. About 99% of the poor (the bottom 10% of the lowest income population) were living in rural areas in 2003.[1]

Economic development in China has undoubtedly had positive effects on health, but along with the large gaps in economic development, disparities in health status and health care have been observed. These disparities arise partially from the persistent urban-rural socio-economic differences, and the problem of lower access to health services by rural households, especially due to financial barriers to access in the form of user fees. In 2002, the maternal and infant mortality rates in rural areas were, respectively, 1.9 and 2.9 times those in urban areas [2]. In 2003, life expectancy of the rural population was about 6 years less than that of urban residents.[1] Additionally, a higher proportion of rural than urban dwellers did not use any health care services when they fell ill.[3] Even for preventive services, the coverage was much lower in rural areas than in cities. For example, the immunization coverage of hepatitis B was about 15% lower in rural areas.[4]

---

1 Division of Primary Care and Maternal and Child Health, Shandong Provincial Department of Health, Jinan, China
2 Center for Health Management and Policy, Shandong University, Jinan, China
3 World Health Organization, China

The rural population spent a higher proportion of their incomes on health care than urban residents and received less government health subsides. In 2003, health care accounted for 13% of total household expenditures in rural areas, which is 4% higher than for urban households.[3] In 2004, the rural population accounted for 58.2% of the total population, but received only 38.6% of total government health expenditures.[5] Rural areas faced greater financial constraints in developing their health care system, as did rural households in accessing health services.

The health situation became a public policy issue after the outbreak of severe acute respiratory syndrome (SARS). At a time when many other Asian countries were making rapid improvements in health and moving towards universal insurance coverage, the World Bank documented the shortcomings of the Chinese health system for the poor, and the 2003 National Health Service Survey (NHSS) showed low health insurance coverage in rural areas.

To improve the health status of the large rural population, the Chinese Government decided to develop a new rural health scheme, the New Cooperative Medical Service (NCMS) scheme, in accordance with the doctrine of building a xiao kiang (well-off) society and achieving greater social justice in health.[6] The NCMS is financed based on health insurance. For the last five years, the NCMS has been accorded high priority from the Government at all levels and has developed rapidly. Following an initial pilot in 257 counties[6] and the scheme's evaluation, in 2007 the Government decided on the goal of achieving NCMS coverage in at least 80% of counties in China by 2008, with 100% coverage in rural areas, and increased the average per capita funding from 30 Yuan (US$ 4.00) to at least 50 Yuan (US$ 6.80).[7]

Because the new rural cooperative medical service system is still at an early stage of development, several problems exist in the process of its implementation. The two most prominent problem areas are the equitability of the system and its management.

1.1 Equity concerns

- **Premium levels:** The current NCMS scheme is strongly supported by government subsidies, with only about 25% of premiums contributed by individual households. However, the total premium level of about only about 50 Yuan per capita is low compared with the high level of medical expenditures. This low level of financing implies limited provision of health care reimbursed by the NCMS. Because of the small reimbursement, the insured still need to spend a lot of money out-of-pocket to receive needed health care. In addition, the NCMS collects premiums from households without regard to their incomes, so the poor and the rich contribute the same amount. This practice has resulted in coverage differences between the poor and rich.[4]
- **Reimbursement:** Due to the relatively low total financing, the reimbursement level is low and out-of-pocket payments remain potentially catastrophic for poor and vulnerable households. In most pilot areas, except in parts of the more economically developed areas of eastern China, the average reimbursement level for those insured by the NCMS is only 20 to 30 Yuan per capita, at the initial stage. In contrast, the 2003 NHSS found that the average expense in rural areas was 91 Yuan and 2,649 Yuan for hospitalization,[4] while the average reimbursement rate for hospitalization fees was only 25.7%.

- **NCMS benefit package:** The current NCMS scheme is focused on curative care, leaving some essential services, including maternal and child health care, outside of the NCMS benefit package. Preventive services are the most cost-effective and would benefit the poor and vulnerable population most because these are currently not provided free of charge. How these services can be included in the NCMS benefit package is an issue directly related to the equitability of the NCMS.
- **Health services use:** One of the principal objectives of NCMS is to increase the use of needed health care services by reducing financial barriers to access for the insured. Studies show that the low-income insured use less inpatient care than the high-income insured.[5] Because NCMS schemes include mechanisms to control moral hazard (such as deductibles, co-insurance, and ceilings), the poor still face financial difficulties in utilizing health care, even if they are insured. This is especially serious if the medical assistance fund (MAF), which operates for the poor independently, does not support NCMS co-payments and deductibles. The MAF is financed by the provincial government budget and managed by the Department of Civil Affairs.

1.2 NCMS management needs to be strengthened

- Shortage of management personnel and funds influence the efficiency of the NCMS. Most NCMS staff can handle only simple, repetitive, daily work and their ability to plan activities, supervise provider behavior, and analyze information remains low.
- Management problems such as complicated reimbursement mechanisms deter the use of needed health services, and failure to control fraudulent use and inefficient provider behavior results in increased costs and reduced benefits.
- The lack of reliable systems to ensure service quality results in lower patient satisfaction levels.[6] Staff have no experience monitoring system performance to check if the poor and vulnerable are receiving their due share of good quality services.

Acknowledging the need for improved policies, Chinese health leaders are now required to enhance the rationality of the health system using evidence based on scientific research. Under this mandate, both researchers and local NCMS implementing agencies in Shandong province wished to look further into the problems and successes of the new system and to improve the policies that govern it. The goal was to improve the equity and efficiency of the NCMS.

The project "Bringing Health Care to the Vulnerable—Developing Equitable and Sustainable Rural Health Insurance in China and Viet Nam" is financially supported by the European Union, with eight participating agencies from Europe, Viet Nam and China. In China, the aim of this four-year project is to improve NCMS design and implementation in terms of equity, quality, and efficiency, through the development and implementation of interventions. Three counties with varying development levels were selected as pilot areas in both Shandong province and Ningxia Hui Autonomous Region. From the beginning, the project emphasized the importance of linking academic researchers with policy-makers in selecting research topics, collecting evidence for developing interventions, and monitoring the implementation of the interventions. Policy-makers involved in this project come from national, provincial, and county levels, providing a good foundation for making the research useful for influencing policies. The project has now finished developing the interventions and is in the process of implementing and monitoring them. The project in Shandong province is discussed in this case study.

> **Shandong province a brief introduction**
>
> Shandong Province is located on the east coast of China and is the second most densely populated province in the country. The total population is 93.09 million, 71.4% of which is rural. There are large regional differences within the province in terms of economic development. The per capita net income of farmers is 4368 Yuan (US$ 595). By the end of March 2007, all 134 counties of the province had established the NCMS, covering 59.9 million farmers, a coverage rate of 90.1%.[6] Although Shandong is advanced in its implementation of the new system, compared with most other provinces in China, it shares the issues mentioned above.

2. The overall process of developing and testing policy changes

2.1 Stakeholders

From the beginning of the project, the academic researchers have accorded top priority to communication with policy-makers. The project team includes central and provincial government policy-makers responsible for the NCMS. Table 1 summarizes the interests and policy-making roles of the various participants in the project.

Table 1: Primary policy-makers and other stakeholders in the project

Stakeholders	Main concerns
Policy-makers	
County health bureau (NCMS office)	• Develop overall design of NCMS scheme • Ensure good health system management • Ensure high coverage rate
General government (Finance bureau)	• Ensure fiscal balance of local finance • Ensure high coverage rate • Ensure satisfaction of rural households
Provincial and central level health policy-makers	• Develop basic guidelines for NCMS policy
Other stakeholders	
Health care providers	• Receive more revenue from NCMS
Beneficiaries	• Obtain more benefits (reimbursement, better quality of care, more convenient reimbursement, etc.) • Receive fair allocation of benefits (especially to the poor)
Academic researchers	• Refine design and implementation of the NCMS scheme • Influence policy-makers to implement recommendations
County Civil Affairs bureau	• Provide financial support for vulnerable population • Help the poor cope with catastrophic health costs

2.2 Stages

The project has included the following stages, from the development of the research proposal to implementation of the interventions:

Figure 1. China Shandong-European Union NCMS Research & Decision Progress

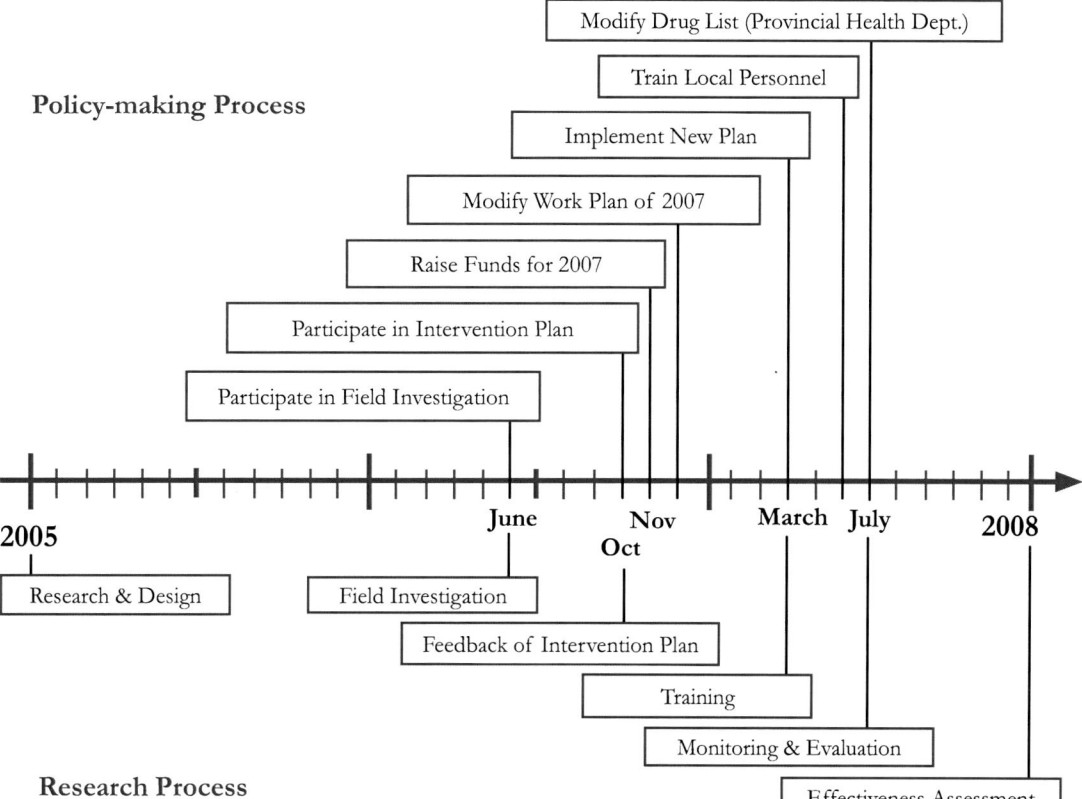

1. **Project launch:** The opening conference was held in October 2005, with central and provincial government health officials participating, as well as those from the pilot counties. Project goals and the implementation plan were thoroughly explained to representatives of the pilot counties in order to gain the commitment of the local policy-makers.
2. **Situation analysis:** A baseline survey was conducted to gather evidence based on which to plan the interventions. Equity issues were included in the survey. Based on questionnaires returned by the pilot counties before the start of the field research in March 2006, the baseline survey was modified so that the study better reflected the needs and willingness of the project counties. After the data collection and analysis, the baseline summary report was prepared in August 2006. Feedback from local stakeholders enabled the researchers to check and supplement the data, and modify the conclusions accordingly.
3. **Design of proposals for interventions:** The intervention design stage was the key stage at which the evidence was used. The research team kept in close contact with the

pilot counties during the intervention plan design process. This process enabled the researchers and policy practitioners to accommodate and understand each other. Repeated discussions with the local population to interpret the data and modify the proposed policy interventions increased their trust in the evidence obtained and in the overall process. In August 2006, a preliminary intervention plan based on the result of the baseline survey and subsequent discussions was distributed to the pilot counties for review. Intervention proposals that elicited the most interest from the local stakeholders and were considered most feasible were written in more detailed and concrete form, including local suggestions. At the annual meeting in September 2006, the research team submitted the intervention plan of the project for discussion and amended it according to the suggestions received.

4. **Discussion of the intervention plan:** It took several rounds of discussions for policy-makers and researchers to agree on the intervention design. In October 2006, a meeting was held with staff from all the project counties. The researchers and policy-makers on the team explained to local officials the content and the evidence base for each proposed intervention, using domestic and foreign experience to support the evidence. Interventions that did not receive full agreement were discussed further. Measures that the participants viewed positively, but considered difficult to implement at the time, were also written into the proposal so they could be reconsidered when conditions permitted.

5. **Presentation of final recommendations to local government:** After receiving the last formal feedback from the pilot counties, at the end of October 2006, the research team submitted the report of the baseline investigation and the amended recommendations of the pilot counties to the Provincial Health Department, for use in formulating the 2007 county health plans.

2.3 Implementation of the intervention package

The intervention implementation stage of the project started in 2007. A strong sense of local responsibility, detailed work plans, and continuous technical and information support were important to the smooth implementation of the intervention plan. Responsibilities were divided among different institutions. The Shandong Provincial Health Department was responsible for direct communication with and supervision of the project counties, and the project counties were responsible for adjustment of policies and methods used to implement the plan. Shandong University was responsible for technical support for implementation. Together with the county implementers, the researchers formulated a timetable and detailed workplans for implementing the interventions in the different project counties.

2.4 Monitoring and evaluation

In April 2007, Shandong University researchers and the Provincial Health Department met with the project counties to develop the monitoring plan. As well as being the basis for the development of the evidence-based policy, monitoring and evaluation were necessary for ensuring timely implementation of the intervention plan, assess project efficiency and equity and make continuous improvements. Indicators for assessing improvement in equity included net reduction of health care costs, health service use, allocation from the Medical Assistance Fund to the poor, and coverage of maternal and child health services. The research team visited the project counties to monitor implementation and prepared quarterly progress reports.

3. How evidence was obtained and used

3.1 Methods used

Zhangqiu, Changle and Donge counties were selected as pilot counties, respectively representing counties of Shandong Province with high, medium and low levels of economic development. Three townships in each county and three villages in each township were further selected by random sampling. The investigation had three parts: the family health survey, the organizational survey and the qualitative investigation.

The family health survey covering 3,339 households and 11,789 individuals using formatted questionnaires was carried out in May and June 2007. Postgraduate students in health management from Shandong and Fudan universities were used as field investigators. The survey included self-reported health status, health service use and expenditure, patients' satisfaction, awareness, knowledge and attitudes about NCMS, and general household characteristics. The survey considered needs of equity analysis by including indicators of income, age, and sex.

The main function of the organizational survey was to assess participation in and cooperation with NCMS by socio-economic dimensions, the NCMS balance of funds, and reimbursement levels, using data such as the volume of services, conditions of providers and fees for services.

The qualitative investigation relied on focus group discussions. The target groups were NCMS policy-makers, administrative staff, community members, and health service providers. The main topics for discussion included understanding of NCMS, the status of its implementation, reasons for the poor not being able to join the NCMS, including financial barriers, and problems experienced and their causes.

3.2 Evidence for design of intervention plan

Based on the analysis of data from the three baseline research components, the researchers selected evidence to design the intervention plan, after verifying it with local staff to ensure its accuracy. The analysis yielded the following findings, which were used to develop the interventions:

- **Discrepancy between individual premium levels and ability to pay:** The 10 Yuan premium contribution from households themselves represents only 0.18 to 0.29% of the average annual per capita net income, which suggested that they are able to pay higher premiums. In addition, the 40 Yuan total premium is only 8% of the average per capita health expenditure. The investigation found that more than 38% of households were willing to pay the 15 to 20 Yuan premium. Considering the steady increase in medical expenses and the likely increased use of services by rural households, financing levels should be steadily increased to avoid a deficit of funds. It is also generally considered that local governments can increase their subsidies.
- **Low level of local government subsidy to the NCMS.** The basic mode of public income redistribution in China occurs at the provincial level, with provincial revenues used

to subsidize county budgets inversely to the ability of local government to raise revenues. Table 2 shows that, in 2006, Shandong province contributed 12 Yuan per capita for the NCMS in Donge county, but only 4 Yuan to Changle and zero to Zhangqiu. This brought the public subsidy part of the total premium to 30 Yuan for all the counties. The central government NCMS subsidy is set at 8 Yuan for all eastern counties having at least a 70% farming population, regardless of economic condition, but increases to 20 Yuan in the poorer counties of the central and western parts of the country.

Table 2: Indicators and premium contributions for sample counties (Yuan) 2006

Indicators	Zhangqiu	Changle	Donge
Per capita net GDP	21 933	12 214	12 701
Per capita income of farmers	5 475	4 565	3 382
Individual premium contribution	10	10	10
Premium as percentage of income	.18%	.21%	.29%
Local government NCMS premium contribution	22	18	6
Provincial government NCMS premium contribution	0	4	16
Central government NCMS premium contribution	8	8	8
Total premium	40	40	40
Per capita medical expenditure	657	475	453

- **Low reimbursement rates:** Using the data on the number of households insured in each income group, the amounts of inpatient services used, and NCMS reimbursement per inpatient, the total reimbursement to each income group was calculated. For all inpatient care, an average of 25.7 Yuan was found to have been reimbursed to the insured. People in the lowest income group received an average of 20.5 Yuan, while in the highest income group each insured person received an average of 38.1 Yuan—nearly double the reimbursement for the lowest income group. The reimbursement rates for hospitalization in county hospitals in Zhangqiu, Changle, and Donge were respectively 18.9%, 15.9% and 4.5%.
- **Failure to protect the poor from catastrophic illness:** The main objective of the NCMS is to protect rural households from catastrophic medical expenses, but the baseline research suggested that it is failing to do this. As Table 3 shows, the proportion of persons insured with catastrophic medical spending (medical spending more than 40% of total household income) for inpatient care varied across income groups. More than 50% of patients in the two lowest income groups had catastrophic inpatient expenses, compared to only 12.5% of patients in the highest income group. In the total insured population, an average of 1.8% had catastrophic medical spending on inpatient care, ranging from 2.8% in the lowest income group to only 0.6% in the highest. Table 4 shows the financial effect of catastrophic expenditures by income groups. Higher income groups had higher inpatient medical expenses, but not proportional to their income. They also received a higher percentage of NCMS reimbursements. As a result, low-income patients actually had a net co-payment that was much higher than their annual income, while for high income patients, the co-payment was lower than their income.

Table 3: Distribution of catastrophic expenditure on medical care

Income group	Number of insured in sample*	Proportion of catastrophic spending among total insured	Proportion of catastrophic spending among total inpatients
I (lowest)	3 724	2.8%	53.8%
II	4 043	2.8%	59.8%
III	4 036	1.6%	32.7%
IV	4 032	1.4%	30.7%
V (highest)	3 930	0.6%	12.5%
All groups	19 765	1.8%	48.1%

*Those with valid information on financial expenditure on inpatient care.

Table 4: Distribution of NCMS reimbursement for catastrophic illness*

Income group	Per capita annual income (Yuan)	Mean expenditure per inpatient** (Yuan)	NCMS reimbursement per inpatient (Yuan)	NCMS reimbursement rate	Co-payment for catastrophic illness as % of annual income
I (lowest)	823.8	2 924.2	369.1	12.6%	330%
II	2 072.8	2 729.5	349.3	12.8%	120%
III	3 175.3	2 450.0	482.6	19.7%	60%
IV	4 750.9	3 907.9	488.7	12.5%	70%
V (highest)	10 863.6	4 391.2	695.8	15.8%	30%
All groups	4 335.1	3 285.7	475.6	14.4%	80%

*For hospitalizations that cost more than 40% of annual income before NCMS reimbursement.
**Direct medical expenses.

- **Lack of financial incentives for using maternal health services:** Maternal health services were not fully used and their reimbursement was very low. Systematic management of pregnancy is a basic component of primary health care. However, because of low awareness by health care providers and low economic status, antenatal management in rural areas was generally worse than in urban areas. In Donge, the average prenatal examination time per pregnant women was only 3.9 minutes compared to the 7 minutes recommended by the Ministry of Health, and the percentage of women who received follow-ups by a doctor after delivery was only 38.3%. In all, only 36.3% of hospital deliveries received NCMS reimbursement.
- **Inadequate management capacity in NCMS.** Each NCMS staff had to manage on average 160,000 participants, with a budget of only 0.1 Yuan per capita. Most staff lacked the skills and experience needed to manage compensation plans and supervise health facilities. At the township level, NCMS was still at the manual operation stage. NCMS organizations were seen as weak in popularizing knowledge about NCMS, providing information, and managing service providers. The rural people themselves were often unaware of how the NCMS worked and what benefits they could receive. Only about 10% of those enrolled were correctly informed about the reimbursement procedures. Many

were unable to get reimbursement as they did not seek service according to the guidelines, and of these, many belonged to disadvantaged groups.
- **Economic barriers:** The poor faced major financial barriers to access to medical services. Of those sampled, 28.6% of respondents could not afford the NCMS premium, while 50% of those who were charged over 10,000 Yuan for hospitalization fell into debt as a result. NCMS is a health insurance system oriented towards households with average incomes and does not provide specific assistance for poor families. This raised the issue of coordination with the Medical Assistance Fund to support premiums and coinsurance payments for the poor, but the fund is the responsibility of the Civil Affairs Bureau, which has little input into NCMS operations and policies.

3.3 Design principles of the intervention plan

To ensure the feasibility of the proposed interventions, the research team adopted the following principles through the design process:
- **Evidence-based principle:** The intervention plan was proposed on the basis of the findings of the baseline investigation. All the proposals were supported by qualitative and quantitative data, as well as by documented experience from other countries. Therefore, local policy-makers understood what needed to be changed, as well as why and how to do so, which facilitated their work and provided them the initiative to implement the interventions.
- **Feasibility principle:** Proposals were developed for the three project counties considering their socio-economic development levels, the human environment, and the level of NCMS development. Proposed interventions were identified for the different counties according to their individual circumstances rather than with the aim of designing a controlled experiment.
- **Multi-sector participation and combination of research and practice:** Local policy-makers from various government departments were involved throughout the process of intervention design, and close contact was maintained. To improve the feasibility of the plan, academic viewpoints were combined with the practical experiences.
- **Equity as a goal:** In the intervention plan, all the suggestions concerning the NCMS were aimed at helping the disadvantaged groups receive adequate NCMS compensation and get equal health services. For example, reimbursement for hospital delivery mainly benefits poorer women, and coordinating the Medical Assistance Fund with the NCMS benefits the poor and vulnerable groups.

3.4 The recommended intervention packages

Based on the above principles, the research team developed the intervention plan with participation of the project counties and international partners. The following recommendations featured in the intervention packages for the project counties.

1. **Increase the level of financing:** Before the intervention, the insurance premium in all three counties was 10 Yuan. The recommendation from the research team was to increase the individual premium in 2008, in Zhangqiu to 20 Yuan, in Changle to between 15 and 20 Yuan, and in Donge to between 15 and 20 Yuan. The policy of provincial and municipal governments is to transfer budget resources from rich areas to poor areas, with local governments in rich areas providing higher subsidies from their own budgets. The total subsidy from the central,

provincial, municipal and local governments was 34 Yuan in Zhangqiu county and 30 Yuan in Changle and Donge, with provincial and municipal government budgets providing 8, 12, and 24 Yuan respectively. The research team recommended increasing the provincial government subsidy to the counties, with more resources going to the poorer counties. The team recommended increasing the local government subsidy to 30 Yuan in Zhangqiu, to between 10 and 20 Yuan in Changle, and to 10 Yuan in Donge. The policy of using the Medical Assistance Fund to subsidize premiums for the poor was recommended for all three counties.

2. **Adjust the benefit package:** Before the interventions were introduced, hospital delivery and maternal and child care services were not included in the benefit package in Zhangqiu and Changle counties. Donge provided a family medical savings account for using outpatient services, with no further reimbursement after the fund was spent. The intervention proposal recommended the inclusion of hospital delivery and systematic maternal and child heath care services in the benefit package. In Donge, the team recommended continued compensation of outpatient fees for those who used up all the funds in their family medical savings account.

3. **Adjust the reimbursement rate and increase reimbursements to the poor:** Before the intervention, the segmented fee schedule in the three countries was typically too complicated and reimbursement rates for the lower fee segments too low. For example, in township centers in Zhangqiu, there was only 20% reimbursement for expenditures between 1000 and 5000 Yuan. The deductible in the county hospital was relatively high in Zhangqiu. In Changle, the reimbursement rate was low in the county hospital, where there were many admissions. There was no deductible for hospitalization in both Changle and Donge, which encouraged many outpatients to try to be admitted as inpatients. The recommendations for all three counties were that the number of fee segments should be reduced, the reimbursement rate should be higher for the lower fee segments, and additional reimbursement to the poor should be provided through the Medical Assistance Fund. It was also suggested that there should be a deductible for hospitalization in Changle and Zhangqiu.

4. **Build management capacity:** Before the intervention, the county NCMS offices had five to seven staff. Although a computer network had been installed, some township level management staff did not know how to use it effectively. Some county level policy-makers lacked sufficient experience in designing reimbursement packages and calculating reimbursement rates. The weak capacity to control the behavior of providers was obvious, and township management personnel and village doctors did not understand the policy well. It was recommended that the number of NCMS management staff be increased and more training given to them and to village doctors.

4. Preliminary evaluation of interventions

4.1 Implementation of recommended intervention packages

According to follow-up investigations by the research team and the Provincial Health Department, most of the proposed interventions were accepted by the local policy-makers and issued as official documents. A few were not implemented, or implemented in a modified manner:

1. **Increases in the level of financing:** There was no increase in individual premiums in the three counties in 2007, although officials in Changle promised to raise them to 15 to 20 Yuan by 2008. In 2007, the provincial government subsidies were increased to 2, 6, and 14 Yuan in the high, middle and low-income areas, respectively, and local government subsidies increased to 40 Yuan in Zhangqiu, 26 Yuan in Changle and 14 Yuan in Donge. The total government subsidy for 2007 therefore increased to 50, 40, and 36 Yuan in the counties respectively. It is expected that the provincial subsidy will be increased further in 2008. The Medical Assistance Fund was implemented to subsidize NCMS premiums for the poor in all three counties.
2. **Adjustments to the benefit package:** The recommendation to include hospital delivery of newborn babies in the NCMS benefit package was implemented in all three counties. The reimbursement rate for hospital deliveries was increased to 30% (higher than for hospitalization for other causes) in Zhangqiu and to 200 Yuan in Changle. Women receiving complete, systematic maternal care in Donge would receive a reimbursement of 100 Yuan, and for hospital delivery, the same reimbursement as for other admissions.
3. **Adjustments to the reimbursement rate schedule:** The fee segmentation was simplified to two to five segments, except in Zhangqui, where the status quo remained. The reimbursement rate was raised in all three counties. In Zhangqiu, both outpatient and inpatient reimbursement was raised by 5%. In Changle, reimbursement for township hospitalization was increased by 10% and for county hospitalization by 5%. In Donge, the reimbursement rate for both outpatients and inpatients went up by 10% and an additional 25% reimbursement for outpatient care was implemented, after the family medical savings account was used up.
4. **Building management capacity:** The research team held a workshop to help improve the management capacity of the county NCMS managers. The NCMS office in each country provided specific NCMS training for township, village and other personnel at least three times. In addition, the NCMS was put on the agenda at the regular monthly meetings of village doctors. Computers are now used in some village clinics.

4.2 Rejected intervention suggestions and reasons for their rejection

Most of the recommendations were accepted by local policy-makers and implemented Some, however, were not taken up.

1. Zhangqiu and Donge counties did not increase the individual premiums. The rate of NCMS participation was an important target and an indicator for evaluating the performance of local officials. Thus, some were concerned that, in the absence of a formal request from higher authorities, increasing the individual premiums would reduce the participation of rural households in the scheme.[4] As the increasing trust of rural households in the NCMS became more evident, NCMS officials became more willing to consider such an increase.
2. Zhangqiu and Changle counties did not adjust the inpatient deductibles. The reason in Changle county was that this might cause dissatisfaction among patients who needed hospitalization. In Zhangqiu, there were technical problems with the computer system.

---

4 Rural households' currently high voluntary participation levels are probably as much due to indirect financial pressures exerted on them by local government, as to the households' own perception of the benefits received

Even though all the recommendations were not implemented immediately, they still had an influence on local policy-makers, several of whom indicated their willingness to increase the individual premiums when most people could really enjoy the benefits from the NCMS. Training also played a significant role in influencing their thinking, with some suggestions that had not been accepted before being put on to the agenda again. For instance, all the three counties expressed that, in the next stage, they would try using NCMS compensation as an incentive to improve patients' compliance in the management of chronic diseases.

While from the beginning, the research enjoyed the participation of local policy-makers, and local social and economic conditions were taken into account, the new policy recommendations still need to be adjusted and improved as the NCMS develops. Some important policy areas were not included in the project, such as whether the NCMS should aim at reducing the financial burden due to rare events of catastrophic disease, or the more frequent burden caused by the basic treatment of common illnesses. In practice, both are targeted at present, but sustainability considerations require a more scientific approach to how NCMS reimbursements should be allocated between the two. This will be on the future research agenda for improving equity through the NCMS.

4.3 The effectiveness of implementation (preliminary observations)

Because the research programme is still in a preliminary phase, it is impossible to do a full evaluation. According to monitoring reports from the project counties, however, the research tem has already observed several positive results.

- In all three counties, the subsidy from the three levels of government was raised by 10 to 14 Yuan and average per capita financing was increased to 50 Yuan.
- Different degrees of reimbursement are now offered for hospital delivery and several families have received these NCMS benefits. In Donge, more pregnant women are using systematic antenatal health care services and receiving reimbursement for them.
- Implementation of the Medical Assistance Fund for the poor population improved the equity effects of the NCMS and health service system. In Zhangqiu and Donge, the amount of funds used in 2007 were higher than in the previous year.
- In Donge, the number of beneficiaries receiving outpatient reimbursement increased by 34% over the previous year.

5. Experiences and lessons learned

There are no final conclusions yet because the project is still ongoing. However, the following experiences and lessons can be summarized based on the work to date.

1. *Close collaboration between the research team and policy-makers is necessary.* The lack of collaboration mechanisms in most policy research projects in China is a primary reason why research results have not had much influence on policy. In this project, the research team worked together with policy-makers from the beginning and good communication among all stakeholders was maintained throughout. This was useful to help policy-makers understand

and participate in the research and helped raise consciousness of their responsibility to implement the interventions. The research team involved policy-makers in the project who had experience both in practice and research, which strengthened both the credibility and feasibility of the findings and interventions.

2. *Attention should be given to the communication strategy.* The research results should be disseminated through effective channels, such as through higher authorities, formal meetings or training courses that attract more attention from participants and can increase their sense of participation. Pedantic and rigid theorizing should be avoided, while communication as between equals is necessary, especially with grass-roots level staff. Policy recommendations should be based on rigorous research but need not be presented in very formal academic language. Researchers should adopt user-friendly language and use both facts and feelings of affinity to reach agreement with local policy-makers.

3. *The research recommendations should be implementable and practical:* For the grassroots policy-makers, conceptual suggestions are not enough: assistance in formulating concrete operational measures is also often necessary. Full consideration should be given to the realities of policy-making and the local environment and training and sustainable technology support are usually needed. It should not be assumed that the baseline survey evidence alone was responsible for the policy changes. The issue of raising the personal premium is an example of how health policy and politics are interlinked in China, as elsewhere, and it is possible that decisions to raise public subsidies also responded to higher-level political pressure.

4. *Timely monitoring and evaluation should be carried out following implementation:* This can especially help local staff to collect information, discover problems and deviations, and offer recommendations for improvement. It demonstrates the sense of responsibility of the researchers and helps facilitate implementation of the new policies.

5. *Research on policy issues should not be a one-time event or relevant to only a single stage of system development.* It should be a high-level, cyclical process, progressing from the adoption of research results into new policy and practice, to the initiation of more and deeper research on emerging issues. Ideally, research should provide continuous support to policy-making.

Acknowledgements

The authors would like to thank the European Union for the grant that supported this project. Collaborators from Liverpool School of Tropical Medicine of the United Kingdom, AOK Company from Germany, Karolinska Institute from Sweden, and Fudan University from China are appreciated for their contributions. Dr Steve Fabricant is specifically acknowledged for his contributions in revising and finalizing the paper.

Endnotes

1. China Development Research Foundation and United Nations Development Programme. *China Human Development Report.* Beijing, China Development Research Foundation, 2005.
2. Li Changming. Ponder and exploration. [M] Jilin Science and Technology Publishing House, 2004.
3. Center for Health Statistics and Information, Ministry of Health. *The National Health Services Survey Report.* Beijing, Ministry of Health, 2003.

4. Sun Xiaojie. Review of reported and actual child immunization programme. *Chinese Journal of Primary Health Care*, 2004, 1874–78.
5. National Health Economics Institute. Report on Health Expenditure Study. Beijing, National Health Economic Institute, 2005.
6. Vice-Premier Wu Yi's Speech at the National NCMS Meeting, Yi'chang, December 2003.
7. Vice-Premier Wu Yi's Speech at the National NCMS Meeting, Xi'an, February 2007.
8. Evaluation Group of NCMS Trials. *China's NCMS in Progress*. Beijing, People's Medical Publishing House, December 2006.
9. Wagstaff A. *et al. Extending health insurance to the rural population: An impact evaluation of China's new cooperative medical scheme*. World Bank Policy Research Paper 4150. Washington, DC, World Bank, 2007.
10. Jiao Y, Sun Q, Meng Q. *Review of CMS in China*. EU project report. Shandong, Shandong University, 2006.

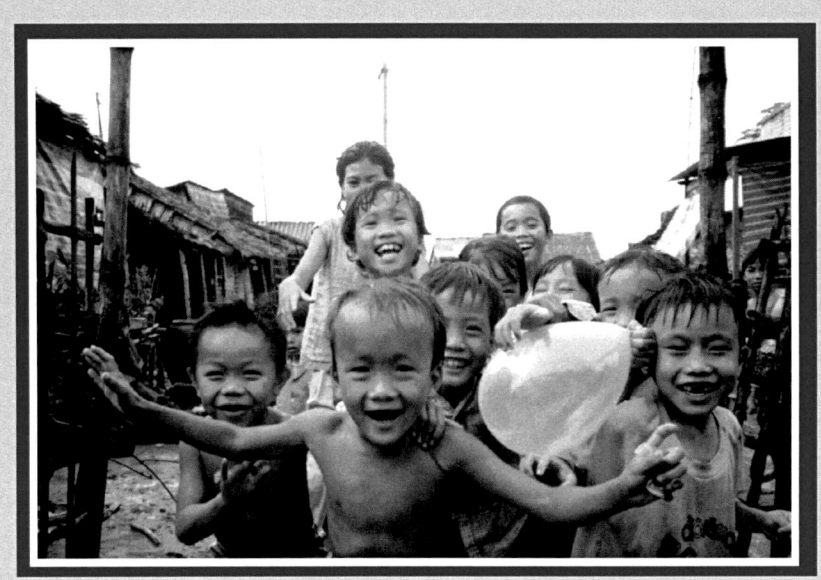

Health Care Fund for the Poor in Viet Nam: how evidence and politics came together

Nguyen Hoang Long[1], Tong Thi Song Huong[1], Dang Boi Huong[1], Tran Thi Mai Oanh[2], Sarah Bales[3], Nguyen Thi Kim Phuong[4], Henrik Axelson[4]

1. Summary

This paper describes the evidence for and process that led to the issuance of Prime Minister's Decision No. 139/2002/QD-TTg on the health care for the poor in Viet Nam. According to the Decision, known as Decision 139 and issued on 15 October 2002, all people identified as poor (based on the national poverty line), are entitled to free health care at public health care facilities and their health care cost is covered by a Health Care Fund for the Poor (HCFP) that is to be established in every province/city and financed by the state budget.

Like other low income countries, Viet Nam faces a shortage of funding for the health care system. Starting in 1989, the Government introduced user fees at public health service facilities, thereby unintentionally making access to health service often unaffordable for the poor. To mitigate the impact of user fees, the Government introduced several policies to partly exempt the poor from payment for health services. However, the effectiveness and the coverage of the exemption policies was very limited, due to inadequate funding and lack of strong political commitment from local government authorities.

During 2001 and 2002, studies were conducted on the use of health services, household expenditure on health, equity in access to health services, and health outcomes. This evidence was well documented and presented in a series of national workshops and forums, which helped to consolidate political commitment among high level government offices, the national assembly and the finance sector to support the poor in paying for health care. At the same time, the grassroots health care system was being strengthened, the national health insurance system was growing, and economic growth provided additional revenues. All these factors together created a synergy which helped influence the highest level of government, and led to Decision 139.

Since the implementation of the Health Care Fund for the Poor in 2003, a number of studies were conducted to monitor and evaluate the programme's impact and give feedback to government policy-making bodies. To further maximize the benefits of the programme to the poor, in 2005, the Government decided to include all the poor into national compulsory health insurance programme, with premiums fully subsidized from the central budget.

---

1 Ministry of Health Viet Nam
2 Health Strategy and Policy Institute Viet Nam
3 Consultant
4 World Health Organization, Viet Nam

2. Introduction and purpose

Starting in the late 1980s, Viet Nam underwent major reforms towards a market economy. User fees at public health facilities were put in place but created major barriers to access to health care, especially for the poor. The Ministry of Health tried to find a policy that could help remove financial barriers for the poor, which would be acceptable to the Ministry of Finance as well as the highest government policy-making bodies.

The Department of Planning of the Ministry of Health sought to convince the Ministry of Finance to adopt a policy to earmark resources to cover the health care costs of the poor. During this process, questions arose about which modes of financing and payment would maximize benefits to the poor.

The latest policy, known as Decision 139 on Health Care for the Poor was proposed and approved by the Prime Minister in 2002. The policy was the result of combining appropriate evidence with strong political efforts. The purpose of this paper is to explain how evidence combined with political factors and contributed to putting this policy in place.

3. Background

3.1 Country context

Viet Nam has a large population of 84 million, living primarily in rural areas. About 14% of the population belongs to one of 53 ethnic minority groups. Population growth has been reduced through an effective population policy and total fertility rates are at replacement levels. Lowering the burden of large family size and of a rapidly growing population have contributed to economic development and poverty reduction (Table 1).

GDP growth has been relatively high and stable since 2000, although half of the population is still employed in low-productivity agriculture. Poverty has fallen dramatically but remains high by international standards. With its rapid rate of development, Viet Nam is expected to graduate from low-income status to become a middle-income country in a few more years.

Currently, Viet Nam's government health services consist of a hierarchy of five levels, starting with village health workers and commune health stations, followed by district and provincial hospitals, and at the highest referral level, the central hospitals. Grassroots-level facilities and workers are widely available throughout the country, ensuring basic primary and preventive health care for all, although the quality of care varies greatly across localities, and tends to be worse in remote and mountainous areas. In addition to the public health sector, the private sector is growing rapidly. Currently, the private sector consists almost entirely of pharmacies and outpatient clinics, although the private hospital sector is growing.

Viet Nam spends about 5% of its GDP on health (2003), which is about average for low- and middle-income countries. However, the public share of total expenditure is only around 30%, making health financing heavily reliant on private expenditure, mainly in the

Table 1: Key statistics of Viet Nam

Population (2006)[a]	84 million
Urban population (2006)[a]	27%
Ethnic minority share (1999)[b]	13.8%
Population growth rate (2006)[a]	1.26%
TFR (2005)[c]	2.1
Real GDP growth (since 2000)[a]	7-8%
GDP per capita (2006)[a]	US$ 722
GDP per capita ($PPP)	US$ 3500
Agricultural share of GDP [a]	20%
Agricultural share of labor force[a]	50%
Poverty rate based on national poverty line (2006)[d]	18.2%
Poverty rate based on $2 a day (2006)[e]	36%
Total health spending (2003)[f]	5.2% of GDP
Public share of total health spending (2003)[f]	29.9%

Note: The poverty line is defined as the minimum level of income deemed necessary to achieve an adequate standard of living. For 2006, the national poverty line, as defined by the government, is VND 200,000 per month for rural areas and VND 260,000 per month for urban areas.
Sources: a General Statistics Office 2007; b General Statistics Office 2000; c General Statistics Office 2006a; d MOLISA; e World Bank; f Ministry of Health 2006.

form of direct out-of-pocket payments by households.[1] This form of payment is seen as the least equitable and creates a substantial barrier to access, especially for the poor. Except for some preventive services, such as the expanded programme on immunization and a few free curative activities such as for tuberculosis and malaria, virtually all health care services require payment, either through prepayment mechanisms, such as contributions to health insurance, or through direct out-of-pocket payment at the time of seeking care. A national health insurance system mainly covers workers in the formal sector, retired government workers, meritorious people, and, from 2006, the poor (estimated at about 20% of the population). For the rest of the population, voluntary health insurance is offered, but the country is still struggling to expand coverage to the entire population.

3.2 Evolution of HCFP policy

The strategy for health care for the poor in Viet Nam has three components. First, the health sector gives high priority to the prevention and treatment of health conditions particularly affecting the poor, e.g., childhood diseases preventable by immunization, tuberculosis, leprosy, malaria, and HIV/AIDS. Second, the health sector has made substantial investments in the health facilities and health workers closest to the population, namely, the village health workers and Commune Health Stations (CHS). Third, the government is trying to ensure the availability of financial assistance to help the poor access curative care. This last component is the focus of this paper.

As Figure 1 shows, Viet Nam has experimented with policies to provide financial assistance to the poor for health care since the reforms that put in place user fees (Decision 45). After a short time, the government realized that the poor were not able to access health care, so exemptions were mandated, but without a clear funding source to compensate facilities (Decree 95). This was also found to be ineffective, as facilities could not exempt people from user fees if their costs were not covered through other funding arrangements.

Figure 1: Timeline of policies on health care for the poor, 1989-2007

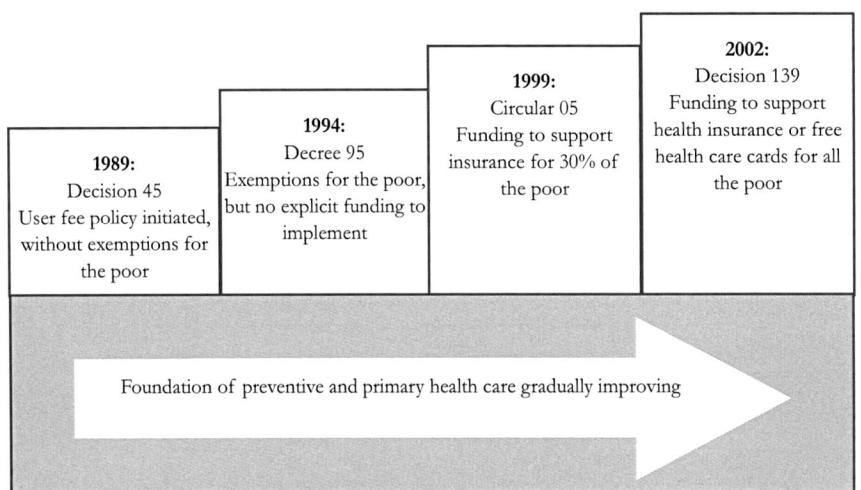

In 1999, Circular 05 mandated government payment of health insurance premiums for the poor, but limited funding permitted coverage of only part of the population. In addition, coverage remained low because provincial budgets were inadequate and the provinces had difficulty identifying the poorest among the poor to receive health insurance or free health care cards (Figure 2). In 2002, by ensuring sufficient funding from central budget sources to cover all of the poor, Decision 139 enabled the Ministry of Health to overcome this serious shortcoming. The next section describes how this important change became possible.

Figure 2: Number of health insurance cards for the poor, 1999-2002

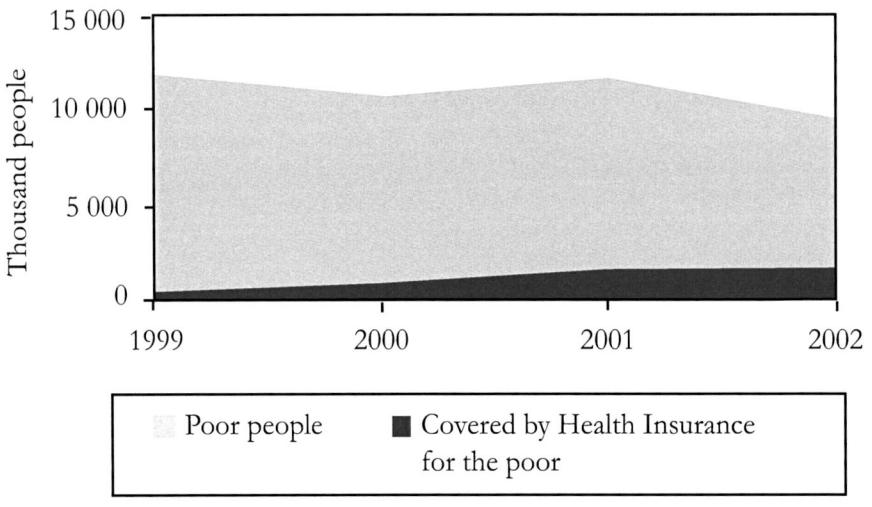

Sources: For poverty rates (percentage of population living on less than 1 PPP$ per day): World Bank (2003); for health insurance coverage: Vietnam Health Insurance Agency, 2002a.

4. Process leading to Decision 139 and health care fund for the poor

4.1 Use of evidence

A variety of studies and reports had a critical impact on the policy-making process leading to the design of the HCFP and the Prime Ministerial Decision 139 of 2002. They are reviewed below.

4.1.1 Evidence on the need for support to the poor

Several qualitative and quantitative studies were conducted on use of and expenditure on health services. One study indicated that illness was one of the most important risks faced by the poor, and led to both a loss of income and high medical costs.[2]. Others indicated a very high financial burden on poor households from user fees at public hospitals.[3,4].

A body of evidence also showed that significant inequalities existed in access to health care and in health outcomes. Using household living standard survey data from 1993 and 1998, a health sector review identified considerable differences across households in various income quintiles with regard to contacts with health services.[3] Figure 3 shows these differences for public hospitals and private clinics in 1998. At the same time, the review revealed that the better-off capture a much larger share than the poor of public subsidies to hospitals. The review also found that inequalities had increased between 1993 and 1998.

The accumulated evidence on inequality was important in the policy process leading up to Decision 139, since it showed that measures needed be taken to provide financial support to the poor to achieve an equitable health system, an important goal of the Government.

Figure 3: Annualized health services contact rates per capita 1998

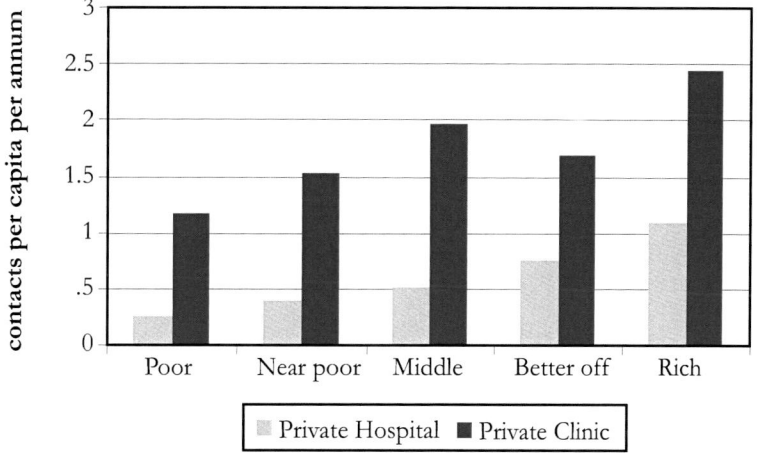

Source: World Bank, 2001

4.1.2 Review of existing policies

Evidence generated from the analysis of previous and existing policies suggested that, despite improvements in the mechanism to provide health care support to the poor, the policy still had many flaws and needed to be substantially strengthened.

- Several studies lent support to the use of health insurance as a mechanism to provide coverage for the poor. Most provincial health bureaus and hospitals supported use of the health insurance mechanism, since it was a major improvement over the former direct reimbursement scheme to support the poor, and in particular, because it guaranteed a payment to the hospital to cover the cost of the care provided.[5]
- The very low enrollment rates of rural residents in voluntary health insurance indicated the limited capacity of the poor to pay their own premiums, thus lending support to the idea of government subsidies.[4]
- Several studies indicated problems resulting from inadequate provincial budgets in poor or remote provinces,[6,7] even though the treasury had adequate resources to compensate. This led provinces to reduce the number of beneficiaries and created disincentives for facilities to treat poor patients.
- Two studies highlighted the fact that the premium for health insurance for the poor was set too low. The actual average health expenditures reimbursed by insurance ranged from VND 34,000 to 75,000 (approximately 16,000 VND to 1 US$), so the premium under Circular 5 of VND 30,000 did not allow Vietnam Health Insurance Agency to cover costs of reimbursing providers.[8,6]

This evidence lent support to the idea that the existing support to the poor under Circular 05 should be expanded through use of health insurance with an adequate premium. It also implied that most of the funds should be provided from the central government budget rather than being an increased burden on provincial budgets.

4.2 Political commitment

A critical enabling factor of Decision 139 and the HCFP was the strong political commitment from the central and local levels to supporting the poor and reducing inequities in health. The National Assembly's Committee on Social Affairs and the Ministry of Health attempted to highlight the issue of the lack of affordability of health care for the poor. In many workshops and meetings the Ministry of Health indicated the political will to: (1) give priority to solving the health problems of the poor, (2) increase access to health care among the poor, (3) reduce the financial burden on the poor resulting from use of health care.

The Communist Party's and Government's strategy of social mobilization ("socialization") emphasizes the political goal of health equity and supports mechanisms to ensure health care for the poor. Government Resolution 90 of 1997 promoted the establishment of funds, with partial financial support from Government, to provide health care for the poor and to enhance the grass-roots health care network. Government Resolution 05 of 2005 on strengthening socialization in education, health, culture and sports added the objectives of: achieving universal health insurance coverage by 2010; increasing the number of facilities allowed to accept insurance reimbursements; and shifting from subsidizing providers towards subsidizing users through health insurance. The goal of universal health insurance coverage was emphasized in several other policy documents as well.

Decree 06 of 2002 of the Central Party Committee on strengthening the grassroots health care network indicated commitment to the importance of basic health care. This reflected concern for the poor because the first contact of the poor when they become ill is normally the Commune Health Station (CHS) or district hospital. The commune health service benchmark (Decision of 370 of 2002) is another step forward by the Ministry of Health to ensure quality of health care at the commune level.

The Ministry of Finance's interest in increasing health spending in a pro-poor direction was an important factor that clinched the agreement for the policy. Growing evidence that the Government was spending too little on health, that its high spending on hospitals was pro-rich, and that hospital autonomy was likely to increase financial barriers to the poor from seeking health care, had put pressure on the Ministry of Finance. Thus, when a proposal was made for the central budget to increase subsidies for health care for the poor, the Ministry of Finance was interested. The crucial compromise was the Ministry of Health agreement to implement hospital autonomy more strongly (with the potential to reduce the financial burden of hospitals on the state budget) in return for the higher premium subsidy for health insurance cards for the poor, thus reducing the concern about the negative impact of hospital autonomy on health equity.

4.3 Enabling factors

In addition to the strong evidence and political commitment in support of the proposed policy (namely, the HCFP), several other enabling factors and circumstances were crucial to the success of passing Decision 139.

One crucial pre-existing condition for rolling out a major assistance programme to provide curative care to the poor in Viet Nam was the existence of a widespread health care system that extended down to the commune level. This ensured that preventive care and public health measures were in place throughout the country, reducing the burden of infectious disease that would have made curative care exceedingly expensive for such a large population and reducing geographic access barriers.

Viet Nam had begun implementing a social health insurance policy since the early 1990s. The Vietnam Health Insurance Agency was under intense pressure to increase coverage of the population and was very amenable to a policy in which the Government would subsidize health insurance cards for people who normally would not be able to afford them. In addition, the existence of mechanisms for issuing cards, verifying patient records and other areas of health insurance administration in all provinces allowed the health care for the poor programme being developed to rely largely on existing structures, rather than having to start from scratch.

The existence of a mechanism for identifying poor households under the Hunger Eradication and Poverty Reduction (HEPR) programme was an important enabling condition that reduced the administrative costs of targeting households under Decision 139.

Rapid economic growth, resulting in increases in budgetary funds available, was a crucial factor that enabled the Ministry of Finance to make the financial commitment needed for Decision 139. Sustainability of funding is considered more likely under government budget financing than if the policy were supported by donors.

4.4 Decision 139: Health Care Fund for the Poor

On October 15, 2002, the Government of Viet Nam promulgated Prime Ministerial Decision 139 on health care for the poor. Under this policy, the provinces would set up health care funds for the poor funded primarily through the Central budget, with the possibility of additional mobilization of funds from the province or other sources. Additionally, the HCFP would purchase health insurance or directly reimburse health facilities for services provided to the poor. Eligible beneficiaries include the poor and some other vulnerable groups. Beneficiaries are to receive the same benefits as the compulsory-insured and measures were put in place to ensure that services were covered from the commune level upwards. The HCFP can also be used to support partial payment of the hospital costs of the near poor facing high healthcare costs in connection with a chronic or catastrophic illness.

The Ministry of Health issued guidelines for the implementation of Decision 139 in 2002. In 2003, most provinces formed management boards and established HCFPs, with the rest completing this task in 2004. In 2005, the Government introduced a new Health Insurance Decree 63, which required, among other changes in general health insurance regulations, that all the HCFP beneficiaries be included in compulsory health insurance. Therefore, since 2005, almost all provinces have adopted the health insurance mechanism to provide financial assistance to the poor for health.

5. Implementation and impact of HCFP

In 2007, the Ministry of Health conducted an impact evaluation study, with technical inputs from international partners. The study examined issues in the implementation process that may have affected impact, including the effectiveness of targeting. The impact on outcomes such as service use, out-of-pocket spending and living standards was analyzed. The findings were checked for consistency with data from the health information system in Viet Nam. Several qualitative studies of Decision 139's impact were also done. Some of the key results from these studies are described in this section. These were used to recommend further HCFP policy improvements.

5.1 Implementation process in the provinces

5.1.1 Findings from analysis of implementation at the provincial level

Although the eligible beneficiaries are clearly specified in Decision 139 and the implementation circular, there were differences across provinces in determining eligibility. Some of the variation was due to logistical issues, but some provinces chose not to cover the non-poor and others used HCFP funds to cover population groups that should be covered under different mechanisms, but which were not adequately funded. This evidence suggested the need for greater clarity in the policy guidelines and to ensure coverage for poor people not officially recognized in HCFPs as such—for example, temporary residents—through an alternative mechanism.

Management boards were required to issue either a health insurance card or a free health care card to the beneficiaries. This proved to be a costly and time-consuming process in some provinces. Studies suggested the need to find a more efficient way to issue the cards, to monitor that cards actually went to the intended beneficiaries, and to ensure an alternative mechanism to provide temporary assistance for people whose cards contained errors or were delayed.

Decision 139 allowed the provinces a choice of provider reimbursement mechanism. The provinces could either purchase health insurance or arrange to directly reimburse providers from the HCFP. Initially, many provinces chose direct reimbursement because of inadequate allocation of funds to purchase health insurance. The variation in reimbursement mechanisms led to misunderstandings and management inefficiencies. In 2005, the new health insurance regulations in Decree 63 stipulated that all HCFP benefits should henceforth be administered through health insurance.

Decision 139 intended to address the constraints of previous policies to finance health care for the poor due to limited funding by ensuring adequate funding from the central level. However, many provinces reported that inadequate allocations from the provincial budget continued to be a problem, leading to under-coverage of eligible beneficiaries. Low disbursement rates were a related problem. On the other hand, many provinces that received adequate funds did not spend all of the funds they had been allocated. At the other extreme, some richer provinces with better medical facilities and high-tech services spent more than the money allocated for the HCFP, with the shortfall made up through the social health insurance fund. These findings suggested the need for stronger measures to ensure that earmarked funds allocated from the central budget are actually used for the intended purpose, and to create the correct incentives and reduce barriers for the province to take advantage of the resources available to help the poor.

Decision 139 encourages use of services at the commune level, but also reimburses the poor when they require paid care at the tertiary level. However, in 2004, a large number of communes were not eligible for health insurance reimbursements, especially in disadvantaged regions. These findings indicated the need to further strengthen the quality of grassroots health service facilities and find a mechanism that allows them to be reimbursed for services provided to the poor even if all the requirements are not met.

At the other end, very few poor people benefited from tertiary level services through HCFP. Only 27 provinces referred Decision 139 beneficiaries to central hospitals in 2004. Of all Decision 139 patients, the total share of inpatients and outpatients visiting central hospitals was only 0.13%. This low rate of referrals for HCFP beneficiaries is partially attributable to the inability of the poor to pay the non-medical costs of seeking care at higher level facilities. Also at play, however, is the fact that the hospital health insurance funds are used to reimburse services for patients they refer to tertiary hospitals, without providing any control over the cost of the services provided. Attempts are being made to create mechanisms to cover the non-medical costs for the poor when referred, but cost control mechanisms for referral hospitals reimbursed by health insurance are not yet in place, creating disincentives for hospitals to refer any insured patients, including the poor.

5.1.2 *Effectiveness of targeting*

After a year of implementation, monitoring showed that under-coverage was a major problem. Nearly half of those from households in the lowest income quintile had not yet received a health insurance card or free health care card by the time of the Viet Nam Living Standard Survey (VHLSS) in 2004. The reasons given by the HCFP management boards were difficulties in identifying those from low-income groups and ensuring that cards were issued and received by beneficiaries. It was, therefore, necessary to follow up the situation with the most recent survey in 2006, which was not published at the time of writing this paper.

Local authorities considered leakage a major concern, and made strong efforts to ensure that better-off people should not receive HCFP benefits. About 22% of cards were issued to people not eligible to receive benefits from the HCFP. When considering only the target group of the poor, 48% of cards were issued to people not in the lowest income quintile. This was due to policy design that included non-poor residents of 135 communes and ethnic minorities in disadvantaged provinces as eligible beneficiaries (Figure 4).

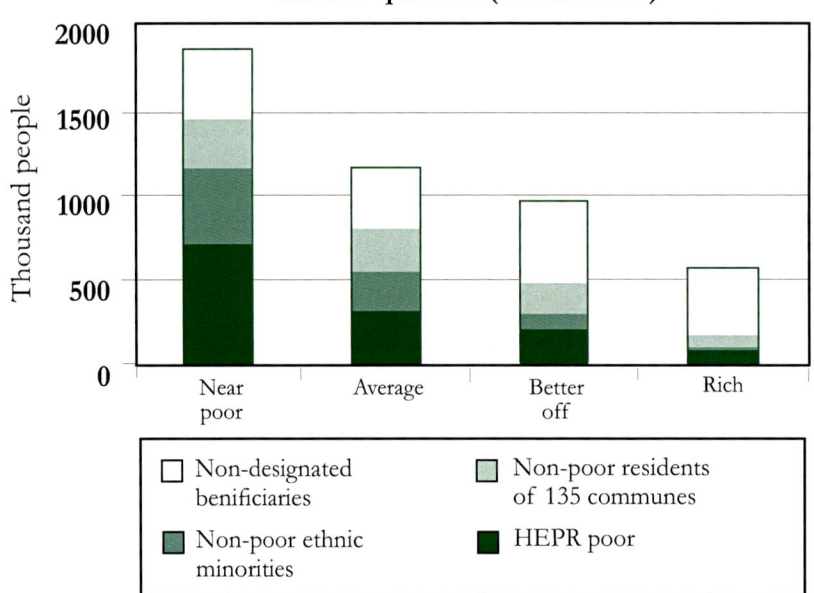

Figure 4: Leakage of HCFP benefits to non-poor, 2004 Income quintiles (VHLSS 2004)

Analysis of targeting effectiveness combined with provincial reports of benefits leaking to the non-poor was useful in considering redefining eligibility of beneficiaries. Under-coverage will decline as the policy becomes institutionalized and issuance of cards becomes a regular activity. The policy will retain the possibility of providing ad hoc assistance for people facing catastrophic health problems who had been missed in the process of identifying beneficiaries. The design of the policy has dropped certain better-off groups from eligibility status.

> **Box 1: Awareness of beneficiaries in Bac Giang and Hai Duong**
>
> Awareness among beneficiaries about the HCFP and its benefits is often weak, as the following quotes show.
>
> "We really lack information about the HCFP. Some people do not know that they need to be provided with health insurance cards because they are poor. Some people who do have the cards do not know what the HCFP benefits are and how they can use the health insurance cards."
>
> "The village leader gave a card to me and he asked me to keep the card for going to health facilities to receive treatment. I was not informed about its benefits. I do not know how the card can be used. I also do not know that we can receive free health care at the CHS. I just found out by chance when I came to CHS to receive treatment."

5.1.3 Awareness of the HCFP among beneficiaries

Awareness by the target population of their eligibility for benefits is a vital indicator to assess if the HCFP functions effectively. Household surveys conducted by the Health Strategy and Policy Institute (HSPI)[9,10] identified reasons why people did not know about the HCFP and why they did not use it if they were insured. They found that as awareness of beneficiaries increased over time, a higher percentage of the target population sought care at public health facilities when they became ill.

5.1.4 Awareness of HCFP among other stakeholders

Awareness of the management board of the HCFP, health workers, health insurance officials, labor officials and commune and village officials is another important indicator of effective implementation of the HCFP policy.

Findings from a 2004 study showed that the policy was effectively disseminated only at the district level. At the commune level, even health workers in some communes reported that they did not know about HCFP policy. A study in 2006 revealed that delays in implementing the policy at the grassroots level could be due to low awareness among stakeholders and officials responsible for implementing the policy. This indicated a need for better information dissemination to all stakeholders.

> **Box 2. Awareness of other stakeholders in Bac Giang and Hai Duong**
>
> The following quotes illustrate levels of awareness about the HCFP among various stakeholders:
>
> "Nobody told us about the HCFP. I never heard its name."
> (A person in charge of hunger elimination and poverty reduction in the commune)
>
> "Even though we are health staff of the Commune Health Station (CHS) who provide health care services, we were not informed that the CHS is responsible for providing health services for insured persons. We only knew when poor persons came to the CHS for consultation and treatment and they told us about it."

5.2 Evidence of impact and outcomes

An impact evaluation using data from the 2002 and 2004 VHLSS found evidence of a positive impact on use of health services by HCFP beneficiaries during the first two years of implementation of the programme. Inpatient service use by beneficiaries was 11% higher than by non-beneficiaries, and 17% higher for outpatient services. Since only state providers could provide benefits during the initial period of the programme, there was an expected shift from private to state providers by beneficiaries. Decision 139 also appears to have reduced self-treatment, as indicated by a reduction in expenditure on self-treatment by households with HCFP beneficiaries.

Province-level data supported these findings. From 2003 to 05, the HCFP contributed to a larger increase in use of services by beneficiaries from poorer provinces than from richer provinces. The consistency of these findings suggests the possibility that the health information system could be used for monitoring this policy rather than more complicated, hard to understand techniques.

In general, out-of-pocket expenditure was reduced, and HCFP beneficiaries spent less than non-beneficiaries on health care. The impact was greater for inpatient care (44% lower for beneficiaries) than outpatient care (4% lower). The HCFP also reduced the incidence of catastrophic spending (defined as spending on health care that amounts to higher than 40% of non-food expenditure), which was 14% lower for beneficiaries.

This early evidence of positive impacts was important in maintaining the political and financial support for continuing the policy.

5.3 Routine monitoring

The HCFP has been monitored since the policy was first implemented. Monitoring has helped to identify problems and shortcomings in implementation as well as several constraints of the current monitoring system, including: delays in reporting, incomplete reports, lack of a clear and consistent monitoring plan with indicators, and lack of cooperation between the various implementing agencies. This indicates the need for clearer allocation of reporting responsibility among the implementing agencies for improving the performance of the HCFP.

6. Revision of policy based on evidence on implementation evaluation of impact

As described, various evaluations have produced a significant amount of evidence on the implementation process and HCFP's impact on outcome indicators, leading to revisions in the policy:

6.1 Recent changes affecting health care for the poor policy

A new poverty threshold was issued in 2005 to ensure that Viet Nam's poverty thresholds meet international definitions. This almost doubled the number of poor between 2004 and 2005. The list of the poor is revised almost every year and HCFP assistance was expanded to include the additional number of poor because funds were considered sufficient to do so.

Decree 63 was issued in 2005, revising the social health insurance regulations. This decree made health insurance for the poor compulsory, with funds to come from the state budget. The package of services covered now includes an expanded list of drugs and diagnostic/treatment services for both poor and non-poor insured. The main impetus for these policy changes was to move towards the political goal of universal health insurance coverage by making it compulsory for additional social groups and by attracting more people to voluntary insurance, but also has clear positive impacts on benefits for the poor.

The Ministry of Finance increased the premium for health insurance for the poor from VND 50,000 per beneficiary to VND 60,000 per beneficiary in 2006 and VND 80,000 per beneficiary in 2007.

6.2 Proposed revisions to Decision 139

The draft of a revision of Decision 139 has been submitted to the Government and is waiting to be approved. The revision will allow the HCFP to reimburse private providers supplying health care to the poor, as long as that they are selected and contracted by a health insurance agency. The original Decision allowed reimbursement of only public providers, which resulted in a shift in health-care seeking by the poor, away from private providers and towards the already overcrowded public sector. There was political pressure to create a level playing field for private providers, and expanding the private sector is seen as a way to reduce the burden of increased use of public sector services.

The new decision also proposes important changes regarding beneficiaries. Non-poor residents of communes categorized as being in difficult circumstances and non-poor ethnic minority people who are almost fully integrated into the national development process are no longer included as beneficiaries. These changes were introduced primarily as a result of political pressure from the provinces that were concerned about leakages to non-poor people inherent in the original HCFP design.

Lack of clarity about eligibility in the original Decision 139 led to a revised provision for assistance to the near-poor (such as non-ethnic minority people living in rural and mountainous regions) in the form of a significant subsidy for voluntary health insurance premiums. Studies using household survey data also produced clear evidence of the need for assistance among the near-poor.

The revision to the policy also allows HCFP to cover expenditures not covered by health insurance to a maximum amount of VND 10 million per episode. HCFP funds can also be used to support treatment costs up to VND 10 million for the uninsured who face sudden difficulties due to high costs.

The earlier policy did not require reporting to the Ministry of Health, but the revised policy makes reporting requirements clearer. Provincial and City People's Committees are required to prepare annual reports to the Ministries of Finance and Health, which will in turn synthesize them into a report to the Government.

7. Conclusions

The Ministry of Health and other stakeholders successfully used evidence (such as evidence on the burden of health care costs for the poor or on inequalities in health care) to convince key government institutions such as the Ministry of Finance that improved and expanded policies to support the poor were needed. The political negotiation process was also important in this regard. Lessons learned from implementing existing policies for the poor were used to design an improved policy.

Another lesson learned from Viet Nam's experience is that once investments in health infrastructure and systems have improved basic health and the country's economy begins to develop, concern can shift toward ensuring health equity in curative and hospital care. If the basic package of primary health care has not been provided, it is inefficient and ineffective to focus efforts and resources on ensuring curative care for the poor as a means to achieving health equity.

Another important lesson is that the HCFP benefited from other pro-poor programmes to assist in identifying beneficiaries. While the identification process is not flawless, the existence of other pro-poor programmes did facilitate the process. Notably, there is political consensus at the central and local levels on which people should benefit from the policy.

Ensuring that free health care cards with correct information actually come into the hands of the poor has been a big challenge. There is, therefore, a need for backup sources of funds for facilities to provide services to people who have not yet received cards, or whose cards contain incorrect information, but who are clearly poor, while improving information systems and perhaps extending the period of validity of the cards.

Ensuring that the poor actually use their health care cards may also be a challenge, if there is discrimination in the provision of services for people with free health care cards. Information dissemination is very important, but must be combined with mechanisms to ensure that the poor are given adequate care.

Guidelines provided to the provincial management boards from the central level were initially not been clear enough for the provinces to implement all aspects of the programme. Recent decentralization of government administration and public finance was intended to allow greater local flexibility in implementing policies and using resources to achieve policy objectives. But when local management capacity is limited, decentralization results in greater need to follow rules given from above, and policies often do not get implemented if those rules are not clear. Written guidelines need to be clear, but also allow for different local conditions. The guidelines need to be accompanied by additional support through field visits and monitoring and evaluation mechanisms.

Funds must actually be disbursed on time and allocated to the insurance implementers in the provinces. There needs to be cooperation between entities at the provincial and district level for monitoring each other and for ensuring that funds are spent correctly.

An important lesson learned from Viet Nam's experience with implementing HCFP is that it is critical to consider and plan for the effects of a new policy on key stakeholders, such as health facilities and the health insurance agency. Many CHS and district hospitals were ill-equipped to deal with the substantial increases in the use of services. In addition, implementation of the policy led to enormous increases in administrative work for health insurance system employees.

Clearly, there are many aspects of the policy that remain to be worked out, and many circumstances particular to Viet Nam. However, the health sector is confident of the direction it is taking to provide health care for the poor, and of its ability to adapt and improve it over time.

Acknowledgements

The authors would like to thank the Government of Cambodia and the WHO Western Pacific Regional Office for hosting the meeting in Phnom Penh and providing a forum in which countries can discuss the use of evidence in designing and implementing programmes that aim to address inequities in health. The authors would like to specifically acknowledge Dr Soe Nyuntu, Ms Anjana Bhushan, Dr Reijo Salmela, and Dr Dorjsuren Bayarsaikhan of the WHO Western Pacific Regional Office and Dr Steve Fabricant, consultant, for their guidance, advice and very helpful comments on earlier drafts of this paper.

The support of the Ministry of Health of Viet Nam to share its experiences with the Health Care Fund for the Poor is gratefully recognized. The authors would also like to acknowledge members of an impact evaluation study that was conducted in 2007, the results of which were used in the development of this case study. Members of the team included Jim Knowles, consultant, Pham Duc Minh and Nguyen Thi Thu Cuc of the Ministry of Health, and Duong Huy Luong and Nguyen Khanh Phuong of the Health Strategy and Policy Institute.

Endnotes

1. Ministry of Health. National Health Accounts implemented in Vietnam for the period 1998-2003. Hanoi, Statistical Publishing House, 2006.
2. World Bank. *Voices of the poor. Synthesis of Participatory Poverty Assessments*. Hanoi, World Bank, 1999.
3. World Bank. *Growing healthy – a review of Vietnam's health sector*. Washington DC, World Bank, 2001.

4. Dong PT, *et al.* (eds.) *User fees, health insurance and utilization of health services.* Hanoi, Ministry of Health, Central Commission for Science and Education, and Vietnam-Sweden Health Cooperation, 2002.
5. Ministry of Health. *Report on user fee implementation.* Hanoi, Department of Therapy, Ministry of Health, 2002b.
6. Akal A. Mission Report to WHO Regional Office and Vietnam Health Insurance Agency on health insurance and financing reform. Hanoi, WHO, 2001.
7. World Bank. *Managing public resources better: public expenditure review.* Joint Report of the Government of Vietnam and the Donor Working Group on Public Expenditure Review. Washington DC, World Bank, 2000.
8. Vietnam Health Insurance. *Report on results of a survey on health care for the poor in 10 provinces.* Hanoi, mimeo, 2002b.
9. Axelson H *et al. The impact of the Health Care Fund for the Poor on poor households in two provinces in Viet Nam.* Paper presented at Forum 9, Global Forum for Health Research, Mumbai, September 12-16, 2005. Hanoi, Health Strategy and Policy Institute and World Health Organization, 2005.
10. Tien TV *et al. Household survey in five HEMA project provinces.* Hanoi, Health Strategy and Policy Institute, 2006.

Additional readings

1. Axelson, H. Impact of Decision 139 on health care utilization: a study using propensity score matching. Background Paper for Workshop on Impact Evaluation of Decision 139, Hanoi, 20 June 2007.
2. Cuc N.T.T., Bales S. Challenges of ensuring effectiveness of Decision 139 under decentralized implementation for the period 2003-2006. Background Paper for Workshop on Impact Evaluation of Decision 139, Hanoi, 20 June 2007.
3. General Statistics Office. *Statistical Yearbook of Vietnam 2006.* Hanoi, Statistical Publishing House, 2007.
4. General Statistics Office. *Main results of the survey of population change and family planning 1/4/2005.* Hanoi, Statistical Publishing House, 2006 a.
5. General Statistics Office. *Results of the survey on household living standards 2004.* Hanoi, Statistical Publishing House, 2006b.
6. General Statistics Office. Microdatabase of the 3% sample of the Census. Hanoi, Central Data processing center of the GSO, 2000.
7. Hung P.M., Dahlgren G., Lieu D.H. Efficient, equity-oriented strategies for health: international perspectives. Melbourne, CIMH, 2000.
8. Huong D.B., Bales S., Knowles J. Implementation of Decision 139: findings from a provincial survey. Background Paper for Workshop on Impact Evaluation of Decision 139, Hanoi, 20 June 2007
9. Luong D.H., Oanh T.T.M. Impact of Decision 139 on living standards of poor households. Background Paper for Workshop on Impact Evaluation of Decision 139, Hanoi, 20 June 2007.
10. Minh P.D. Impact of Decision 139 on out-of-pocket spending of poor households. Background Paper for Workshop on Impact Evaluation of Decision 139, Hanoi, 20 June 2007.
11. Ministry of Health. *Review of options for securing funds for the health care needs of the poor and other groups exempted and reduced from user fees.* Hanoi, National Health Support Project, Ministry of Health, 2000.
12. Ministry of Health. Proposal to Prime Minister to request issuing the Decision on Health Care Fund for the Poor. Hanoi, Ministry of Health, 2002a.
13. Ministry of Health. *Final report of the Vietnam National Health Survey 2002.* Hanoi, Ministry of Health, 2003.

14. Ministry of Health and Hanoi Medical University. *Review of use and provision of health care services for the poor through a survey on discharged patients in some hospital in 10 provinces.* Hanoi, Department of Therapy, Ministry of Health, and Public Health Faculty, HMU, 2002.
15. Vietnam Health Insurance. Health insurance statistical yearbook 1993-2002. Hanoi, Statistical Publishing House, 2002a.

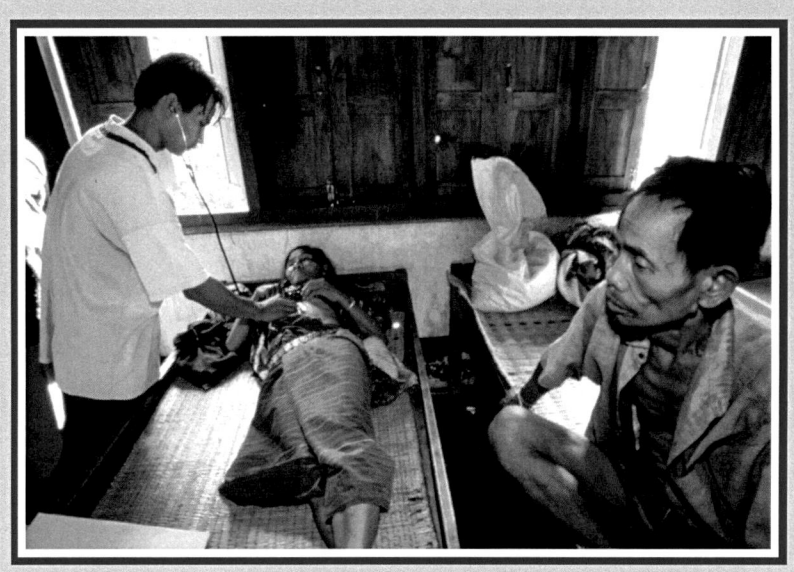

Scaling up primary health care in the Lao People's Democratic Republic using evidence from a long-term primary health care development project

Carol Perks[1], Dr. Khamla Phouthonesy[2], and Dr. Steve Fabricant[3]

1. Summary

From 1992 to 2006, the Ministry of Health in the Lao People's Democratic Republic and the Sayaboury provincial health department implemented a primary health care (PHC) development project in this previously underserved, ethnically and linguistically diverse region in the northern part of the country. A non-governmental organization (NGO), Save the Children Australia (SCA), provided technical advice and support, with AusAID funding. Progress was steady throughout the four expansion phases of the project, and the province now enjoys health indicators equal to those in more developed countries. Detailed evaluations of the project, carried out in 1998 and 2004, showed evidence of great progress and identified reasons for the success of many project activities.

In contrast to most health development projects in the Lao People's Democratic Republic, the Sayaboury project was a "bottom-up" process. The lessons learned were carefully documented, and are the basis of this case study. Key to the success of the project were a constant focus on the community and its needs, the recognition of traditional practices and cultural and language differences, and outreach to remote communities. Although successful outcomes were known and disseminated as early as 1998, another attempt to apply the same approach to primary health care development in the Lao People's Democratic Republic was not initiated until 2006. This paper examines the evidence that replicable and sustainable health improvements were achieved at low cost, how the evidence was used, and its applicability for large-scale health sector development projects.

The health sector in the Lao People's Democratic Republic depends heavily on external donor support. The larger donors support in multi-sector economic development and poverty reduction efforts and, therefore, have significant influence on health policy at the central level. In some countries, sector-wide approaches (SWAps) have improved donor coordination and produced a single approach to primary health care development, but this has not happened in the Lao People's Democratic Republic. The influence of NGOs and other lobbies for the community-focused primary health care approach are weak compared to the large donors.

The major donor-supported projects are usually large in scale, but, due to relatively slow decentralization in health, planning and management skills are stronger in the central Ministry of Health and, to some degree, at provincial level. These projects therefore use a "top down"

---
1 Save the Children Australia, The Lao People's Democratic Republic
2 The Lao People's Democratic Republic Ministry of Health, Sayaboury Province
3 WHO/WPRO consultant

approach, mainly supplying infrastructure and equipment, reinforcing central and provincial-level management, and supplementing funding for vertical programmes.

Even some countries without formal SWAps, such as Cambodia, have achieved agreement between donors and governments on policy and joint funding of primary health care development pilots, with local and international NGOs continuing to play a major role in primary health care projects working at district and village level. Initial doubts about the replicability of the approach used in Sayaboury were reduced as new local NGOs sprang up in response to the availability of donor funds. Although the community-focused approach requires long-term commitments and attention to primary health care principles, its alternative—the "top-down" capital-intensive approach—does not guarantee that improved outcomes will be seen quickly either.

2. Background and health policy in the Lao People's Democratic Republic

The Lao People's Democratic Republic is one of the least developed and poorest countries in the world. In 2002, the infant mortality rate was more than three times higher than that in neighbouring Thailand and Viet Nam, and the fertility rate was more than twice that of its neighbours. The maternal mortality ratio was approximately 405 per 100 000 live births[1] compared with 44 in Thailand and 130 in Viet Nam. Highland ethnic minority groups tend to do less well than the majority population with respect to these indicators.

Many recent improvements in health outcomes can be credited to the establishment of an accessible health delivery service (see Table 1). According to data from the 1995 and 2005 censuses and the 2000 health survey, the under-five mortality rate declined from 170 per 1,000 live births in 1990 to 98 in 2005,[2] while the maternal mortality ratio declined from 750 to 405 per 100,000 live births. Life expectancy has risen to 63 years in 2005 from 45 in 1985, mortality for malaria has been reduced by 60% in rural areas since 1996, and access to clean water has increased from 31.8% in 1995 to 43% in 2004.[3] The trend in the prevalence of undernutrition is uncertain, but undernutrition is currently estimated to affect 30% of children under five.

The Lao People's Democratic Republic is gradually adopting a market-oriented economy, with fairly good economic growth, except in the aftermath of the 1997 Asian financial crisis. The use of health services, a general proxy indicator for improvement of health services and patient satisfaction, has increased, but not at the pace that might have been expected from the investment in expanding the network of health services. In the rugged, mountainous areas of the country, the health of those living in rural and remote villages is further challenged by limited access to the benefits of economic development and to social services. Most households in the 72 poor districts and 47 poorest districts consist of subsistence farmers living in rural and remote villages. The income gap and the health disparities between urban and rural populations are increasing. As many as 76% of the villages and 50% of households are considered poor and lacking in essential services.[4]

The public sector faces considerable governance challenges in ensuring the efficient use of health service resources. The World Bank's public expenditure review for the Lao People's Democratic Republic (2002) identifies the critical underfunding of the health sector, and in particular, the low funding of recurrent expenditures as a major issue. Moreover, health expenditure accounting needs to be strengthened and made more transparent. Current total health expenditure is estimated at 3.9% of gross domestic product (GDP) or US$ 17 per person per year, with 60 to 80% of this taking the form of out-of-pocket expenditure incurred at the time of service.[5]

A system of primary health care based on village cooperatives existed in the Lao People's Democratic Republic even prior to the Alma Ata conference. However, national strategies were not always carefully planned, leading to the dominance of rather verticalized disease control programmes, a situation that still poses a challenge to the effective coordination of primary health care.[6] From 1980 to 2001, four national health meetings were held to evaluate previous performance and plan future operations, resulting eventually in the first National Policy on Primary Health Care in January 2000. The policy recognizes primary health care as the most cost-effective approach for addressing common health problems of the rural poor, in particular women and children.

The Health Sector Strategy to the Year 2020 is a key policy document (see Box 1). The policy for primary health care is based on a high degree of decentralization, which gives provincial-level administration the key role in the implementation of health care services. The central Ministry of Health is responsible for health sector planning, policy development, coordination, external financing and evaluation, while the provincial and lower levels are responsible for strategy development, planning, budgeting and implementation. A Steering Committee coordinates and supervises donor-assisted projects. Provincial primary health care coordination units have been established, sitting at a high level in the provincial structures, immediately below the provincial health officer. The higher status accorded to primary health care coordination should allow improved coordination of all primary health care components, even if they are currently being funded through more vertical and centralized structures.

Box 1: Basic Concepts for Health Development Strategies to Year 2020

The Health Strategy to 2020 has emphasized the following four basic concepts, which will be used to guide future health development efforts:

- Equity of Healthcare Services
- Early Integration of Healthcare Services
- Demand-Based Healthcare Services
- Self-reliant Healthcare Services

Six Major Directions for Health Development to the Year 2020

The Health Strategy to 2020 stresses six directions for health development:
- To strengthen the capability of health staff in terms of attitudes, ethics and technical skills in order to ensure high quality services;
- To improve community-based health promotion and disease prevention;
- To improve and expand hospital services at all levels and in remote areas;
- To promote utilization of traditional medicine by integrating modern and traditional care;
- To promote scientific and research activities for health development;
- To ensure effective health management, including administration, finance and health insurance systems.

Source: JICA Master Plan for Lao PDR

The Ministry of Health has developed an organizational structure, system design, policies and plans relatively quickly. At the provincial level, planning, budgeting, and other management skills have been upgraded. Most provinces have well-trained staff and new primary health care management systems. Decentralization should, in theory, improve the efficiency and effectiveness of services, but core interventions are still delivered through vertical programmes that are centrally managed and do not always integrate well with provincial services. With the gradual devolution of administrative authority, districts are responsible for planning and budgeting. Newly-decentralized provincial and district health offices are struggling to cope with their increased technical and management responsibilities. [7]

The district health system has three main components: the district health service, the community, and village-level health providers. The district health service consists of the district health office, district hospital, health centers, and community-level health workers. [8] Decentralization is intended to help build community participation and self-reliance and ensure that services are demand-driven. However, poorer provinces have sometimes been at a disadvantage following decentralization, as central level resources were cut off.

By the late 1990s, difficulties in access at peripheral levels, low levels of effective demand for services (that is, need for services, backed by economic buying power) and the poor quality of services were recognized as issues to be addressed. Several approaches were proposed, including mobile clinics, shifting more qualified providers to health posts and organizing drug revolving funds (DRFs) where they did not exist.[9] The recent Ministry of Health/Japan International Cooperation Agency (JICA) Master Plan study still found these issues in 2001:

> "Due to the shortage of budgets and staff, district health offices and health centers rarely deliver substantive health services to villages other than some vertical programmes... Even in those vertical programmes, some health staff do not have the requisite communication skills, and they do not conduct activities together with villagers in an interactive manner. People's participation is generally weak in the health sector, with the exception of some donor projects."[10]

The Master Plan identified another general issue that poses a challenge to the success of primary health care in the Lao People's Democratic Republic:

> "Although the central government has the stated goal of securing access of minority people to health services even in remote areas, the same types of programmes and strategies are promoted throughout the country. Such undifferentiated or non-strategic approaches are neither realistic nor effective in providing basic health services to remote areas. Approaches or strategies specially designed for remote areas are required."

Although the Sayaboury Project began a decade before the above observations were recorded, it has focused its interventions on these issues and raised demand by improving quality and meeting the needs of the population.

3. The Sayaboury project

A remote mountainous province on the western side of the Mekong River, Sayaboury Province had a population of 321,000 in 2003. It shares a long border with Thailand and 22% of the population belongs to 33 ethnic minorities. In 1991, Save the Children Australia (SCA) began working with the Provincial Health Office in a setting of inadequate infrastructure, difficult transportation and communications, and isolated and under-trained health staff.

The first steps in building the health system were to strengthen the provincial and district hospitals by training health staff, and provide the necessary infrastructure, equipment and essential drugs. A functional system was necessary so patients and staff could be referred from the village level with confidence. Maternal and child health services were used as an entry point for strengthening other primary health care services.[11] The first phase focused on strengthening the skills of the provincial management team, which conducted training for district teams and dispensary staff, and trained village health volunteers (VHVs) and traditional birth attendants (TBAs). Fixed and mobile maternal and child health clinics were developed, dispensaries constructed or upgraded, and essential equipment provided. District mobile health teams visited each village at least twice a year to provide health education in local languages, and also provided curative care, antenatal care, immunization, family planning and growth monitoring. District teams conducted quarterly "Health Days" at each dispensary, monitoring the quality of services, conducting training, and providing clinical services.

During the second phase, the programme expanded into four additional districts and focused on integrating primary health care activities. District hospitals were provided with equipment and training to improve the quality of referral services and their capacity to support village-level activities. Seed capital and training in the management of DRFs were provided at district and dispensary level. A health information system and routine monitoring and evaluation framework were developed, including six quality indicators.

The third phase expanded into four newly-created remote districts in the north of the province. The fourth phase aimed to strengthen the skills of health workers, especially in the new districts. Training was mostly conducted in the Lao language, and was complemented by training inputs from the SCA advisor and others, study tours, postgraduate public health courses and clinical placements in Vientiane and Thailand. The Integrated Management of Childhood Illness strategy was adopted in all the districts. Studies showed high prevalence of nutrition-related conditions in children, which became a focus of preventive activities and health education.

4. Developing evidence that the programme was effective

The programme was evaluated in early 2004 by the provincial management team and an external evaluation adviser. The assessment used a variety of methods, including the following:

- Reports and documents, in English and in Lao, were reviewed, including Health Data Summaries (1997–2003) and Six-Monthly Primary Health Care Activity Reports.

- Participatory evaluation workshops were held, in which four domains of change were examined: district capacity, provincial management capacity, quality of health services including community perceptions, and impact on population health.
- Impact data from the routine health information system were reviewed for 1997–2003 as were findings from the 1999, 2001 and 2004 population surveys in the northern districts. Some data derived from the health information system were considered possibly inaccurate, especially reporting of births and deaths, since there is no vital registration system, and had to be verified independently.

The primary health care programme achieved significant gains when compared with national health indicators (see Table 1). Provincial health services expanded to include 69 dispensaries delivering clinical services and community-based health promotion services. By 2003, 92% of households in the province were living within 5 km or 60 minutes' walk from a health facility. Improvements in access were accompanied by a tripling of the use of outpatient services between 1997 and 2003. The facility use rate in 2003 (392 per 1000 population) was more than double the national rate.

Table 1. Key health indicators in Sayaboury Province (2003) compared with national data from the Lao People's Democratic Republic (Lao PDR) (2002)

Indicator	Sayaboury (2003)	Lao PDR (2002)
Life expectancy (both sexes)	71 years	59 years
Crude mortality rate	3.3 per 1000 population	6.3 per 1000 population
Crude birth rate	23 per 1000 population	34 per 1000 population
Infant mortality rate	23 per 1000 live births	82 per 1000 live births
Under-5 mortality	29 per 1000 live births	106 per 1000 live births
Maternal mortality ratio	110/100 000 live births	530 per 100 000 live births

Source: Perks *et al.* Bulletin of the World Health Organization, February 2006, 84 2.

The province-wide under-five mortality rate in 2003 was 29 per 1000 live births and the infant mortality rate was 23 per 1000 live births, compared with national rates of 107 and 82. The infant mortality rate was 21 per 1000 live births, down from 47 per 1000 live births in 1999. This low reported infant mortality rate was confirmed by a population survey in the four northern (least developed) districts in 2004.

The proportion of pregnant women having at least three antenatal clinic visits increased from 24% in 1997 to 58% in 2003, compared with 20% nationwide. Training and supervision of TBAs led to an increase in attended deliveries in the northern districts, from 17% of births in 1999 to 47% in 2004. Moreover, all district hospitals in the province were now able to provide basic emergency obstetric care. The maternal mortality ratio decreased from 218 per 100 000 live births (probably under-reported) in 1998 to 110 in 2003, compared with 530 nationally. Given that 86% of women delivered at home and comprehensive emergency obstetric care was not available in most district hospitals, the reduction was attributed to greater birth spacing, good coverage of antenatal care, the training of TBAs, high rates of attended deliveries, and the availability of basic emergency obstetric care.

The decline in mortality is consistent with lower morbidity and improved health behaviours. Reported cases of malaria have steadily declined since 1998. In 2003, 73% of households used an impregnated bednet (compared with 24% nationally), and mortality from malaria had decreased from 15.8 per 100 000 in 1995 to 2.5 in 2003. Significant improvements were observed in infant feeding practices, with 63% of mothers giving their children oral rehydration solution during diarrhoea episodes in 2004.

5. Influencing primary health care policy

The 1999 evaluation described the issues addressed and the lessons learned in establishing primary health care in Sayaboury over an eight-year period. SCA and the Australian Agency for International Development (AusAID) disseminated the approaches and successes of the project within the Lao People's Democratic Republic and the development community.

The issues and lessons drawn from the Primary Health Care Project in Sayaboury are interrelated:
- A project management team approach evolved from a small number of counterparts working with an expatriate advisor. This greatly strengthened teamwork and fostered communication and cooperation between the provincial and district levels.
- Long-term assistance and personal continuity of assistance resulted in a good understanding of the project and contributed to good relationships among all stakeholders. Long-term commitment is required by the implementing and funding agencies.
- All project activities were implemented by government staff, with technical and resource support from SCA. Developing this effective partnership between government agencies and external partners also requires a long-term approach.
- Strengthening capacity at the provincial and district levels at the same time ensured that each level understood the other's role and functions in the system. Before primary health care services could be effectively implemented, a functioning health system had to be operating at all levels. This allowed outreach services to operate and TBAs and VHVs to refer patients to them.
- The formation of primary health care committees within the provincial and district level health departments increased communication and cooperation among health staff, serving in practice to functionally integrate vertical programmes at and below those levels. Intersectoral committees were also instrumental in bringing about cooperation between the health sector and other government departments in the province.
- The heads of each section of the health department (maternal and child health tuberculosis, the expanded programme on immunization [EPI], water and sanitation, health education, malaria, food and drug, and hospital sections) met monthly to discuss issues and solve problems. Terms of reference were developed for the primary health care committee so that all members understood their roles.
- Technical assistance and long-term relationships between government and external partners: Staff of the SCA Vientiane office and the office in Australia provided technical assistance and were responsive to suggestions for changes in activities and reallocation of funds. Health department staff worked closely with an expatriate health advisor resided in the province. This was crucial to capacity building in management and technical areas.

- The primary health care directors and the expatriate health advisor consistently aimed at integrating project activities into the normal routine work of the health department. This was initially a difficult concept for staff, who tended to regard the project activities as separate from their routine work.
- The Ministry of Health monitored project activities and impacts at regular intervals, provided feedback and encouragement to the provincial department of health and to SCA, and helped to share the experiences of the project with other provinces.
- Staff received training in the maintenance and repair of equipment because budgets were limited and this helped reduce the financial burden of replacing equipment.
- District-level staff were not provided with salary supplements, but were given accommodation and food allowances consistent with national government rates.

In summary, the Sayaboury programme benefited from the long-term stability of provincial primary health care leadership, appropriate technical assistance and consistent donor support. Its significant achievements were realized with a modest investment of around US$ 4.3 million over a 14-year period, or only US$ 1.00 per person per year. A study in 2003 found that the recurrent costs of the programme (mobile clinics, health days, monitoring and supervision, three-monthly intersectoral and project management meetings, and annual refresher training for village health volunteers and traditional birth attendants) amounted to US$ 41 000, or less than US$ 0.13 per person per year.

A brochure was written by SCA after the first major evaluation especially to disseminate the experiences to provincial health departments, Ministry of Health and agencies working in the health sector with the Government. It concluded:

"The Government needs to make a conscious effort to analyze and incorporate lessons learnt from district-focused projects. Other provinces would benefit if the Ministry of Health in the Lao People's Democratic Republic were to adopt the district level health management tools developed in Sayaboury and apply them elsewhere, most critically in the 47 poorest districts targeted by the National Growth and Poverty Eradication Strategy."

6. How the evidence was used

Modest inputs, over a prolonged period of time and with a focused and consistent primary health care strategy and vision, yielded good results. The Ministry of Health indicated its support for the Primary Health Care project in Sayaboury, viewing it as a model for how cost-effective primary health care services can be developed and carried out by government health workers. Given the urgent health needs in rural areas, it was expected that this evidence would result in similar approaches being implemented in other underserved provinces. Possible reasons why this did not happen for a long time include the following:

- The statistical evidence of success was seen to be weak. For example, maternal mortality was lower than the national rates but could not be compared to a baseline rate in the province. Even if there had been a baseline rate, it would have been difficult to estimate how much of the reduction was attributable to the intervention and how much to the overall socioeconomic improvement in the Lao People's Democratic Republic, which has experienced steady growth recently. While growth rates in most rural areas were probably

far less than the average 7% for the Lao People's Democratic Republic as a whole, Sayaboury's proximity to Thailand has made it relatively well-off for the area.
- Cross-border ties are often important in the Lao People's Democratic Republic. In Sayaboury, in particular, the issue of higher quality health services available across the border (in Thailand) may be of some importance, especially on an affordable co-payment level under the Thai "30-baht scheme". (This is a reasonable hypothesis for curative treatment, but it seems unlikely that women would travel far for the preventive care that produced the most improvement.)
- The careful and intensive inputs from the NGO and its advisor were key to the accomplishments made by the project. The point can be made that SCA in effect subsidized the project in important non-monetary ways that are impossible to quantify, and perhaps even less possible to replicate.
- Some large potential donors such as AusAID, SIDA and GTZ have recently pulled out of the health sector in the Lao People's Democratic Republic. SCA approached the Ministry of Health at several junctures, but, while supportive, it had no funds to replicate the project.

7. Eventual replication in Nan province

SCA sought funding to replicate the Sayaboury programme in another province for several years without success. Eventually, a small budget was granted by the Korean Government to replicate this project in Nan District, Luang Prabang Province, where health indicators had been worse than the national average.

Commencing in February of 2007, implementation o this replication project has been rapid. In the first six months, use rates at the district hospital increased 44% for outpatient services, 72% for inpatient services and 40% for hospital deliveries. This has been due to the strengthening of district health management systems, improvements in the health facilities, in-service training, provision of medical equipment and supplementation of the essential drug funds with emergency obstetric drugs and rabies and tetanus vaccines.

8. Discussion: government, external donors, NGOs, and primary health care development

The health sector in the Lao People's Democratic Republic still depends significantly on external assistance. The early 1990s saw a rapid increase in foreign funding to health, much of which focused on rural areas where the lack of health services after the collapse of the communes was felt most strongly. The large number of small projects led to many individual initiatives using different strategies, posing enormous challenges for the Ministry of Health's efforts to incorporate them under the umbrella of a national primary health care strategy.

Donor coordination in the Lao People's Democratic Republic is still limited, with Japan's development assistance agency playing a crucial role. JICA funded the Lao Health Master Planning Study in 2001/2002, which identified sector-wide coordination and primary health care as top priorities. Thirty "very high priority programmes" were selected to promote the overall basic strategies (see Annex), including three primary health care programmes, one of which focuses on district health services. As described in the master plan study Executive Summary:

> **PH-3: Implementing the PHC Approach to Strengthen District Health Systems**
> ... aims at strengthening the four components of a district health system: the district hospital-based services, outreach services, health center-based services, and community-based activities. The district is where the top and bottom meet, where policy becomes reality. PH-1 transforms the "Policy on Primary Health Care" into the "Ministry of Health Strategic Plan to Operationalise"; PH-2 lays down flexible national guidelines and regulations, and PH-3 describes activities to actually strengthen the four components... It underscores rationalizing and clarifying the organization, improving management systems, and building capacities of staff to take a holistic approach. It emphasizes the empowerment of communities to take responsibility for their own health. PH-3 proposes the participation of NGOs or consultancy groups as catalyst of change in implementing PHC."

Although the Master Plan identifies an important role for village-level primary health care, it does not go into any detail as to how these functions are to be developed. While it is excellent and comprehensive in most other respects, the Master Plan neglects to clearly recommend a role for NGOs in influencing policy-making at the highest levels or in primary health care implementation. The detailed description of the Plan's primary health care programme in Chapter 14 makes no mention of a role for NGOs. NGOs are mentioned as a possible partner only in Chapter 15 on maternal and child health, and then only cursorily (see Annex).

Although many donors recognize the importance of improving primary health care, their support often takes the form of building capacity and infrastructure, which may also not target villages that are under-served. The Asian Development Bank (ADB) funded a primary health care project in two provinces (which ended in 2000), followed by a large primary healthc are Expansion Project in eight northern provinces, which also strengthened provincial health management nationwide. The World Bank is undertaking complementary primary health care development in the other provinces. JICA and the bilateral cooperation agencies of Belgium and Luxembourg provide support to several model districts.

In some countries, a sector-wide approach (SWAp) has improved donor coordination and generated a unified approach to primary health care development, but this has just begun in the Lao People's Democratic Republic. There is agreement that it is premature for the Lao People's Democratic Republic to use the SWAp mechanism to improve donor coordination and policy implementation. According to ADB:[12]

> "Given the state of public sector financial management and donor coordination, a sector-wide assistance approach would be premature at this time. However, by regular policy dialogue aimed at fostering a common assistance agenda in PHC and communicable disease control, ADB hopes to contribute to a more consistent, coherent and effective utilization of external assistance to the health sector."

SWAps do not guarantee better aid effectiveness and, even in some countries without formal SWAps, donors and the Government have agreed on joint funding and common strategies for health sector development projects. For example, in Cambodia local and international NGOs play a major role in primary health care projects working at district level, using a 'sector-wide management' approach. The initial round of contracting of district health services in Cambodia involved only international NGOs, but initial doubts about replicability disappeared as local NGOs sprang up in response to the availability of donor funds for the second round. Although the community-focused approach to primary health care development is lengthy, its alternative—the "top-down" capital-intensive approach—does not necessarily guarantee quickly improved outcomes either. However, NGO presence and influence are still relatively weak in the Lao People's Democratic Republic and other mechanisms for promoting and implementing community-focused primary health care are lacking.[13] Furthermore, the large health sector donors are more influential.

9. Major donors' approaches to health sector and primary health care development

The current Lao People's Democratic Republic national 5-year development plan (6th Socio-economic Development Plan, or SEDP6) identifies the health sector as one of four priority areas for poverty reduction. The Government is committed to achieving health for all and aims to provide all citizens with access to primary health care. The 5-year plan includes the National Growth and Poverty Eradication Strategy (NGPES), which focuses on the poorest districts. The large donors participate in multi-sector economic development and poverty reduction efforts, and they have much influence at the central health policy level. The lead international funding agencies in the health sector are ADB, the Global Fund to fight AIDS, Tuberculosis and Malaria (the Global Fund), JICA, and the World Bank. The Governments of Belgium, China, India, Luxembourg, and the Republic of Korea also provide assistance.

The NGPES is currently being costed, with initial estimates suggesting a 43% increase in current spending for its full implementation. Within the framework of the SEDP6, the Ministry of Health has prepared a budget of US$ 322 million for 2006–2010, for which it is seeking assistance.[14] (The Master Plan has not yet been completely harmonized with the Health Strategy, and presumably has not been costed yet.) Funds on this scale are available only from the development banks and major donors.

Major donors' projects are usually large in scale, and focus on investments in infrastructure and 'capacity building' in management-related areas and financing. This approach is conditioned by donors' past experiences in the Lao People's Democratic Republic and elsewhere. Most bilateral donors, development banks, and the Global Fund are required to do elaborate preparatory analyses and go through many stages of consultation and approval. Expensive technical assistance is usually needed, often to prepare a plan for further assistance in sector development and capacity building. For example, a recent preparatory study provided US$ 700,000 to:[15]

> "… assist the Government to prepare a plan to improve health sector financing, human resource development, and primary health care. This will include a series of sector interventions aimed at improving the institutional framework, financing, human resource development, and governance in the health sector."

Such high initial overhead costs are justified if large scale projects are planned and money can be disbursed quickly. Even when scaled down to the small population of the Lao People's

Democratic Republic, the large donors' projects tend to dwarf any that could be proposed by even the largest international NGOs. At the same time, economies of scale accrue to the Ministry of Health by having to manage a few large projects instead of many small ones; if the NGPES were to be executed with small NGO-type projects, the US$ 322 million would fund more than 200 projects on the scale of the Sayaboury project for the Ministry to oversee.

Decentralization in the health sector has been slow (and somewhat ineffective, by one large donor's own assessment), so planning and management skills still reside largely at the central Ministry level and to some degree at the provincial level. Absorptive capacity and management concerns may dictate a "top-down" strategy, mainly supplying infrastructure and equipment, reinforcing central and provincial-level management, strengthening specific vertical programmes, and specific, quantifiable, policy areas such as financing. This can be considered "selective primary health care", in contrast to "comprehensive primary health care."[16]

Large donor-financed development projects in health are designed and implemented similarly in nearly all developing countries. In large top-down projects there is often little discussion of activities or investments below the district level:

"... will be implemented by the MOH through its relevant departments and Directorates, and executed by a PMU [project management unit] (at the central level), and Provincial and District Health Management Units (PPMU, DPMU) at their respective levels. A Steering Committee will be responsible for project oversight, and the PMU will report to Ministry of Health's Department of Planning and Budgeting. The main functions of the Provincial PMU include direction and oversight of the Project's district-level implementation, especially the district plans, training quality and effectiveness, as well as monitoring and evaluation. The DPMU's principal responsibilities include district planning, project implementation, including supervision and monitoring of all project activities, and financial management."[17]

While the following project description seems to leave room for NGOs, it would be unusual for a large-scale project to reach below the district level even if its goal is to improve primary health care:

" ... the Project will invest in the development of district health systems, building management and technical capacity for planning and service delivery at the district and provincial levels in a decentralized system. The focus on district planning provides ... a capacity building method which has proved effective in a variety of settings. It will support the efforts towards the integration of vertical programmes through district and provincial management of health services, building on successful efforts by bilaterals and NGOs, as well as coordinating efforts with partners in response to limited government capacity."[18]

10. NGOs in the Lao People's Democratic Republic

Recent data show only 70 international NGOs operating in the Lao People's Democratic Republic, with a total of 237 projects in all sectors. An official decree[19] provides formal recognition to international NGOs and regulates their structure and activities. Notwithstanding recent developments in the private sector, the Government continues to play a key role in economic and social affairs. Although local NGOs have not emerged in the Lao People's

Democratic Republic, mass organizations play important roles in delivering social programmes, as in Viet Nam.

In contrast, as of 2002, Cambodia had over 200 international NGOs and some 400 local NGOs and other registered charitable associations. Their total financial contribution was nearly US$ 100 million, with 15% of all NGO projects being in health. Some 13 000 Cambodians are employed in the NGO sector. Over 40 NGO sectoral and issue working groups, both formal and informal, come together in support of development. Informal NGO networks exist in almost every province and contribute to dialogue on development processes and policies.

Neighboring Cambodia and Viet Nam are also recipients of large amounts of development assistance from bilateral and multilateral agencies and channeled through international NGOs. In the Lao People's Democratic Republic and Viet Nam, the international NGOs work with the mass organizations, while in Cambodia the international NGOs work either directly with communities or in partnership with emerging local NGOs. Donor's suggestions in the Lao People's Democratic Republic to develop local institutions as grant recipients may lead to increased awareness of the possible role of the NGO sector.

Policy-makers' perceptions of NGOs may also be influenced negatively by the work of NGOs in neighboring countries, particularly in Thailand, where NGOs have been vocal in the support of political reform.[20]

11. Conclusions

The Ministry of Health can make better use of available resources and experience in scaling up effective primary health care. There was some debate over the quality of evidence that the Sayaboury project improved health outcomes, and also as to the replicability of the NGO's long-term technical assistance and community-focused approach. For reasons discussed, the Government continues to rely more on the large donors to fund projects that use most of their available resources to address deficiencies in the health system from the top down.

Analysis of how inputs are nominally allocated in the two approaches points to a natural complementarity between them. There cannot be effective primary health care if community-based elements are ignored. At the same time, evidence suggests that large investments in health systems cannot be effective unless management capacity and resources exist at all levels of the system. Balanced capacity at all levels of the health system is necessary. Figure 1 shows that a health system needs both top-down capacity-building **and** the community-focused primary health care strategy. It illustrates the complementarity of capacity-building and community-based approaches at all levels of the health system. For example, even in an isolated environment such as Sayaboury, the primary health care project depended on critical inputs from the provincial and central levels. The project might not have achieved high birth spacing, to which it attributes a major role in reducing maternal mortality, without an effective national family planning programme. Conversely, when the EPI programme in the Lao People's Democratic Republic faced grave challenges due to management and logistical problems, local immunization rates dropped sharply.

Figure 1: Complementarity between top-down and bottom up approaches

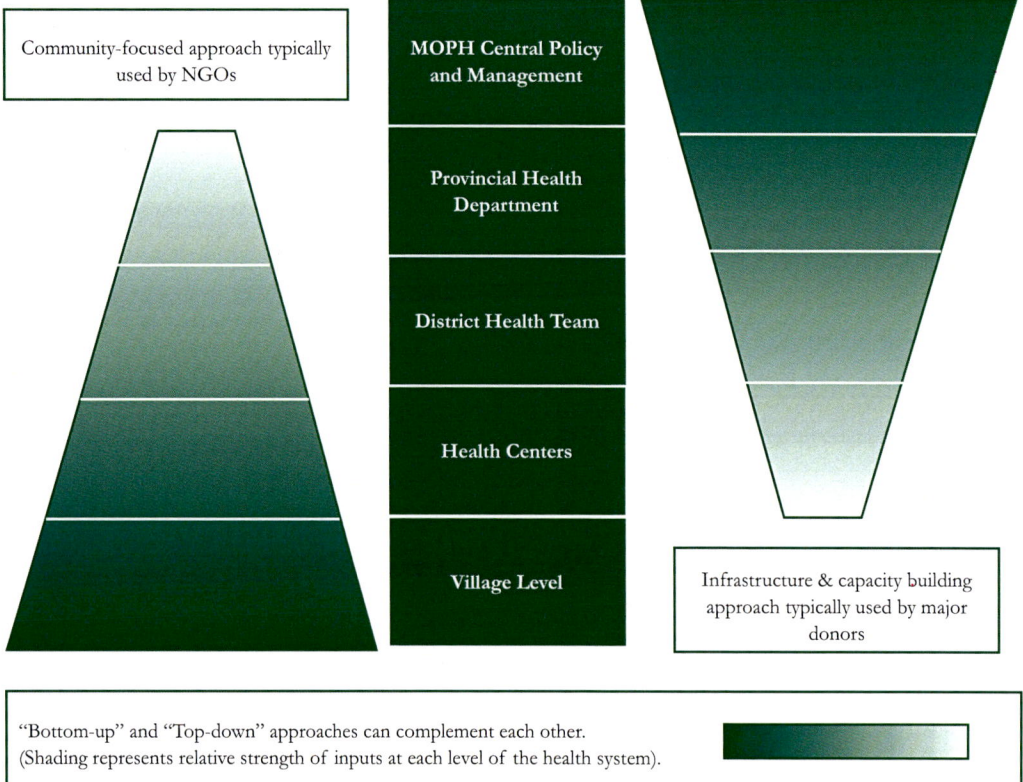

"Bottom-up" and "Top-down" approaches can complement each other.
(Shading represents relative strength of inputs at each level of the health system).

It would be helpful if the recommendation for NGO participation in primary health care development in the Master Plan were stronger. Nevertheless, the Government and other health sector partners in the Lao People's Democratic Republic could consider the Sayaboury project as a balanced, community-based approach to primary health care development.

While a formal SWAp will probably take time, donors in the Lao People's Democratic Republic do not seem to be opposed to sector-wide management arrangements such as are now used in Cambodia, where donor funds are used to contract NGOs to implement primary health care at district and community level. The Master Plan for the Lao People's Democratic Republic accurately identifies the core issues, and it is also very clear from various project documents that the large donors understand these issues well, e.g.:

"The national PHC policy has noticeably broadened the outreach of public health activities and sharpened the focus on sub-District heath centers and VHV but there is still a tendency to focus primarily on infrastructure development at the District/sub-District level rather than the village level (home to the majority of the Lao population) and the bias towards vertical programming remains strong throughout the country. Programmes such as malaria control and EPI are implemented in highly centralized ways that receive specific financial support in the form of per diems for local staff. In contrast, routine PHC outreach tasks are given low priority by lower level health staff largely due to inadequate budgets."[21]

Effective health sector development, however, will require that primary health care at community level is scaled up, with support for the key roles of local organizations and motivators. This case study suggests that the primary health care system which evolved in Sayaboury Province is appropriate for the Lao situation. With commitment, it might not be difficult to replicate this experience in other provinces, as now demonstrated by continued work in Nan District.

References

1. National Statistical Center. 2005 Population Census. Vientiane, National Statistical Center, 2006.
2. *Ibid.*
3. WHO/UNICEF Joint Monitoring Programme in Water and Sanitation. *Meeting the MDGs in drinking water and sanitation.* Geneva, WHO/UNICEF, 2006.
4. Carol Perks, Michael J. Toole, Khamla Phouthonesy. District health programmes and health-sector reform: case study in the Lao People's Democratic Republic. *Bulletin of the World Health Organization*, Feb. 2006, 84 (2).
5. WHOSIS 2004 data.
6. Norwegian Church Aid. Evaluation of HIV/AIDS Program, Lao People's Democratic Republic. Vientiane, Norwegian Church Aid, 2005.
7. Asian Development Bank. 31348-01 Lao People's Democratic Republic Primary Health Care Expansion Project, updated December 2006. Manila, ADB, 2006, available at: http://www.adb.org/Documents/Profiles/LOAN/31348013.ASP, (accessed 12 January 2009).
8. Japan International Cooperation Agency. Lao People's Democratic Republic Health Master Plan, Chapter 14: PHC. Vientiane, JICA, 2001.
9. Ogawa S. *et al.* Unbalanced distribution of health sector human resources and malfunctioning of peripheral health services in Lao PDR. *Ryukyu Medical Journal*, 1998, 18(4):135-141.
10. Lao Health Master Planning Study Final Report, Volume 1: Summary.
11. *Op.cit.* reference 4.
12. Asian Development Bank. *Op. cit.* reference 7.
13. Lyttleton, C. *Cross-border health in the Mekong Subregion: Perspectives from Lao PDR.* Consultant's report. Rockefeller Foundation, 2004.
14. World Health Organization Western Pacific Regional Office. PHC Review Project Region Specific Report. Manila, WHO/WPRO, 2002.
15. Asian Development Bank Request for Proposal, 2005.
16. Lesley Magnussen, John Ehiri and Pauline Jolly. Comprehensive versus selective primary health care: lessons for global health policy. *Health Affairs,* 2004, 23(3):167-176.
17. World Bank. Project Information Document (PID) Appraisal Stage Report No.: AB981, Health Services Improvement Project (HSIP), Ministry of Health, Lao People's Democratic Republic. Washington DC, World Bank, 16 August 2005.
18. *Op.cit.*
19. Lao People's Democratic Republic Prime Minister's Office No. 7 1 /PM Decree of the Prime Minister on the Administration of Non-Governmental Organizations in the Lao People's Democratic Republic.
20. Asian Institute of Technology. Capacity building of non-governmental organisations in Cambodia, Laos, and Vietnam. Project Proposal. Bangkok, School of Environment, Resources and Development, Asian Institute of Technology Bangkok, May 1998.
21. Asian Development Bank. *Op. cit.* reference 7.

Annex

Master Plan Executive Summary

Objectives:
1. To promote sector-wide coordination at national, provincial and district levels;
2. To reform the health financial system and to strengthen the financial management capacity of MOH, provincial health offices, and district health offices;
3. To improve the quality of health worker training, especially of nurses, and to allocate and motivate well-trained health workers in districts and health centres;
4. To build the system and capacity of health management in a decentralised context;
5. To promote efficient and effective infectious disease control;
6. To implement the PHC approach to strengthen district health systems;
7. To operate central and provincial hospitals efficiently; and
8. To increase the availability and affordability of essential drugs and to promote rational drug use.

PH-1 Programme for Supporting the Operationalization of the "Policy of Primary Health Care" PH-1 takes the Primary Health Care Policy another step further towards full operationalization in the Lao People's Democratic Republic. Considering that the developmental approach of PHC is a paradigm shift from the welfare approach, it recommends a re-orientation of attitudes of decision-makers at the central Ministry of Health, PHO, and DHO as well as those of the provincial and district governors, after which the process of formulating the "Ministry of Health Strategic Plan to Operationalize PHC" commence.

PH-2 Programme to Develop and Adapt Flexible National Guidelines and Regulations for Strengthening District Health Systems based on the PHC Approach
PH-2 aims at supporting and facilitating the strengthening of District Health Systems based on the PHC approach by providing flexible national guidelines and regulations. The guidelines/regulations cover the following components of the District Health Systems: 1) District health offices and district hospitals, 2) District health committees, 3) Health centers and health centre networks, 4) VHVs/TBAs and VHV/TBA networks, 5) Village Health Committees, 6) Village Health Providers. PH-2 is identified as a "precedent" programme that should be implemented immediately to lay the foundation for further development.

PH-3 Programme of Implementing the PHC Approach to Strengthen District Health Systems
PH-3 aims at strengthening the four components of a district health system: the district hospital-based services, outreach services, health centre-based services, and community-based activities. The district is where the top and bottom meet, where policy becomes reality. Whereas PH-1 transforms the "Policy on Primary Health Care" into the "MOH Strategic Plan to Operationalize PHC", and PH-2 lays down flexible national guidelines and regulations, PH-3 describes activities to actually strengthen the four components of a district health system: the district hospital based services, outreach services from the district level, health centre based services, and community-based activities of village health volunteers. It underscores the importance of rationalizing and clarifying the organization, improving management systems, and building capacities of staff to be generalists and take a holistic approach. It emphasizes the empowerment of communities to take responsibility for their own health. PH-3 proposes the participation of NGOs or consultancy groups as catalyst of change in implementing PHC.

To Implement the PHC Approach to Strengthen District Health Systems
- To take the following preparatory steps for beginning the development of District Health Systems based on the PHC approach:

- To diffuse the PHC approach at the national, provincial and district levels, and
- To establish flexible national guidelines and regulations for developing District Health Systems according to the PHC approach.

- At the same time, to make the following efforts at reforming existing vertical programmes, existing health centres, village-level RDFs, and district hospitals for preparing for the future development of district health systems based on the PHC approach.
  - To decentralize the planning and management of vertical programmes of EPI, malaria control, reproductive health, water and sanitation, and TB control to the district and, in some cases, to health centre levels,
  - To promote the horizontal integration of these health activities with other health activities at the district and health centre levels,
  - To actively promote activities of MCH, nutrition and health education at first in vertical ways, and then to integrate these activities into the District Health System covering health centres and villages,
  - To rationalize existing health centres and integrate them into the District Health System,
  - To promote village-level RDFs under the effective guidance of district health officers or health centre staff, and
  - To improve district hospitals so as to attract local people and to establish district hospitals/district health offices as the central bases of District Health Systems.

From Chapter 15 on MCH:

"Securing a strong foothold in the critical steps needs the support and assistance of NGOs, UN agencies and other external donors... UNICEF and Non-government Organizations (NGO) may be in the best positions to find approaches on how to implement the package of services in the field…. It is important that the outputs of these critical steps are processed, applied and eventually incorporated into regular MCH activities and services for the entire country."

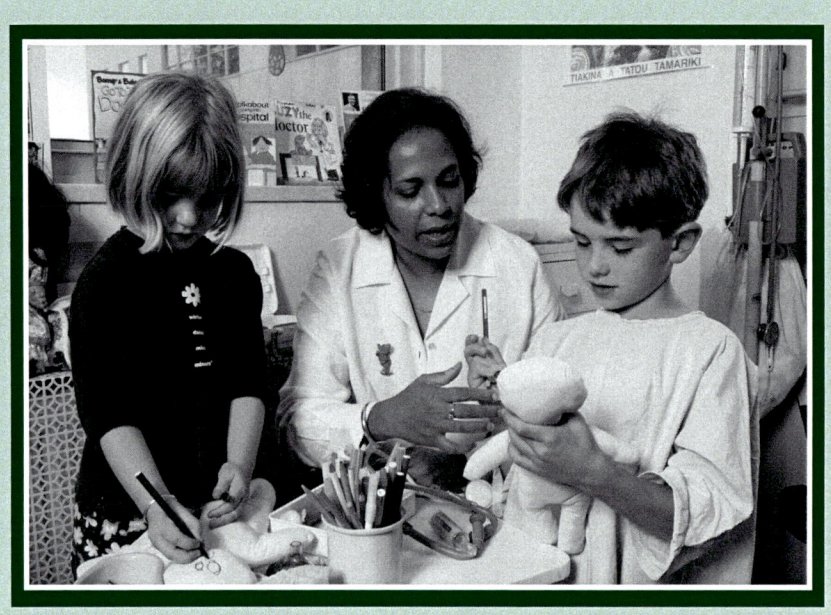

Promoting health equity: evidence, policy and action— The New Zealand experience

Don Matheson[1], Kumanan Rasanathan[2], Martin Tobias[1]

1. Summary

In the last decade, the response to social and health inequalities has moved to the centre of the policy environment in New Zealand. From an absence of general discussion about disparities between groups, awareness has increased to the extent that inequalities are now a significant part of the political debate for the major political parties and central to the policy development and monitoring frameworks, particularly in the health sector. This paper considers how this development has occurred with regard to health and presents initial indicators of the progress made, exploring why New Zealand chose to act on health inequalities and how this has been implemented.

The paper provides a brief overview of health inequalities in New Zealand, followed by a discussion of relevant local literature and tools to address inequalities. It discusses in more detail the development of primary health care as an integral part of the response to addressing health inequalities and a housing initiative as an example of intersectoral action. These developments have occurred alongside changes in other sectors.

The paper concludes with a consideration of the impact of the policy attention to inequalities and further challenges for New Zealand to continue progress in this area.

2. Problem definition

The central question that this paper addresses is whether the actions of the state and other players can reverse an established trend of increasing health inequalities.

The term 'inequalities in health' as used in New Zealand carries connotations of socially-produced disparities that are unfair. Such disparities might be described as 'health inequities' in other regions. In this sense, the New Zealand usage is similar to that in Europe.[1] Throughout this paper, 'inequalities in health' and 'health inequalities' are used in this way, reflecting the New Zealand context. Health equity in the New Zealand context includes but goes beyond equal access to health services to address avoidable and remedial differences between population groups.

---

1 Ministry of Health, New Zealand
2 University of Auckland

3. Assumptions

The underlying assumption is that health improves if a wide range of societal measures are addressed, including wider health determinants (such as income, housing, education, and employment), improved access to health care services, and improved healthy environment, which has a positive impact on tobacco and alcohol use, as well as on food, nutrition and physical activity.

4. Recent history of inequalities in health in New Zealand

Ethnic inequalities have been a focus of the research on health inequalities in New Zealand over the last 20 years. Analysis has been made possible by the National Health Index (a unique identifier for individuals in the health system), greater attention to the measurement of ethnicity in the health sector and new tools such as the linking of census data to health records.

Māori, the indigenous people of New Zealand, have generally worse health status than non-Māori New Zealanders across almost all health indicators. For example, the gap in life expectancy between Māori and non-Māori men is eight years, while that between Māori and non-Māori women is nine years.[2] Māori have poorer access to health services, poorer quality of care within the health system and worse health outcomes for most disease groups.[3]

It is estimated that at least half of the life expectancy gap between Māori and non-Māori is explained by socio-economic disparities, as Māori are over-represented in low socio-economic groups.[4] However, new evidence shows that Māori generally have poorer health compared to non-Māori of similar socio-economic status. Further, Māori in high socio-economic groups have shorter life expectancies than non-Māori in low socio-economic groups.[5,6] Differences in smoking rates explain around 10% of the mortality gap.[7] The experience of racial discrimination (both inside and outside of the health sector) and related poorer access to and quality of health and other services are postulated to explain most of the remaining life expectancy gap.[8,9]

Other minority groups, such as Pacific[10] peoples living in New Zealand, also experience poorer health than the majority New Zealand-European population. Asian[11] peoples in New Zealand comprise almost one-tenth of the population, but show a paradoxical picture in terms of health status, due to the 'healthy migrant' phenomenon.[12,13]

Socio-economic health inequalities have also been well investigated in New Zealand.[14,15] Major inequalities exist and these widened following the economic structural reforms of the 1980s and early 1990s (as described below). The gaps in life expectancy between people from households in the poorest and richest income quintiles are about 9 years for men and 7 years for women.[14] Socio-economic gradients are seen for all ethnic groups in New Zealand.[15]

Other dimensions of health inequalities, such as sex and geography have received less attention in New Zealand. Geographical influences are mediated by the socio-economic and ethnic inequalities described above, but also by differential access to services and health selective migration, as in other countries.[16]

In summary, detailed evidence is now available in New Zealand about health inequalities in terms of ethnicity and socio-economic status. The development of this evidence base over the last twenty years has influenced health policy in New Zealand to the extent that it is now common to plan and monitor health programmes considering these inequalities. The next section of this paper considers how this evidence base was developed and what impacts and interactions it has had with the health policy environment in New Zealand.

5. Prevailing political climate and agenda setting

Health inequalities are now a priority for health sector planning in New Zealand, as well as a key focus in overall social policy. Legislative and policy instruments license and enforce this focus and tools have been developed to increase awareness and workforce capacity to take action on these disparities. Increased recognition of the Treaty of Waitangi (the compact between the indigenous Māori and European settlers signed in 1840) and a growing research base about Māori health have fostered active discussion in academic and policy circles about the historical and contemporary contextual factors responsible for maintaining Māori health inequalities.[17-19]

The emergence of a strong focus on health inequalities can be conceptualized in terms of the different but intersecting public, political and organizational discourses around disparities in health. The public discourse in New Zealand originated from increasing concern in the 1990s around socio-economic inequalities and the threats to social cohesion that these posed. A strong egalitarian value system had operated in New Zealand with respect to fairness of opportunity and lack of hierarchy, arising from a settler culture and New Zealand's revolutionary suffrage movements (New Zealand being the first nation to grant women the right to vote in 1893) and social welfare programmes of the 1890s and 1930s. This belief in equality often failed, however, to recognize the severe impact of colonization on Māori. The structural reforms of the 1980s and 1990s disproportionately affected Māori and also affected Pacific peoples. Mounting anxieties about increased crime rates, poor economic performance and greater cultural diversity interacted with starkly rising inequalities to undermine the sense of egalitarianism by the end of these structural reforms. There was also public unease that the reforms had undermined the egalitarian ideal and greatly increased inequality.

This public concern about unfairness and the impact on inequality of the structural reforms to subsidies, the labour market, public housing and benefit payments created a space in the political discourse for attention to inequalities in health, building on the growing international and local literature. In its third term (1996-1999), the government of the National Party saw the emergence on the political agenda of the health needs of disadvantaged groups, as it tempered its market reforms of the early 1990s (which themselves built on the market and social sector reforms of the previous Labour Government from 1984 onwards). One outcome of this was strong government support for the delivery of health services outside of the mainstream by Māori and Pacific providers.

An important milestone was the publication in 1998 of a report by the National Health Committee (NHC) entitled The Social, Cultural and Economic Determinants of Health in New Zealand.[20] The NHC is an independent statutory committee appointed by the Minister of Health and mandated to provide independent advice to the Minister on health and disability issues. The NHC report brought the issue of health inequalities into the health policy arena (including identifying that inequalities were worsening). Moreover, it provided a rationale for acting on these disparities and recommended actions, including intersectoral action and better access to primary health care. A parallel development during the 1990s was the development of a methodology to describe socio-economic inequalities in New Zealand, the New Zealand Deprivation Index.[21] The Index structured and boosted interest in socio-economic inequalities in New Zealand and provided social agencies with a tool for more closely aligning resource allocation to need.

The new Labour Government—which came to power in 1999 with a strong platform of increasing public spending in health and education, and a policy agenda of "closing the gaps" between the disadvantaged and the privileged in New Zealand society—further built upon the prevailing public and political discourse.[22] The Government implemented new health legislation and began planning a series of health strategies to be developed by the Ministry of Health. The New Zealand Public Health and Disability Act 2000 comprehensively reformed the New Zealand health sector, instituting a population health focus and explicitly requiring the health sector to reduce health inequalities. The key functional documents of Ministry of Health, such as its Statement of Intent and annual performance reviews, now incorporated clear reference to the need for action on health inequalities.

The new Act also reconstituted the funding and delivery of health services by devolving responsibility for local health planning and services to 21 regional health authorities called District Health Boards. These boards were mandated to respond to health needs of their communities and reduce disparities in health status. As a result, a health inequality focus was embedded into the design and delivery of all health services, from preventive to tertiary, at least at the policy level.

Alongside this reorientation in the policy environment was an explosion in the local academic literature on health inequalities. Two key reference works were published by the Ministry of Health: Social Inequalities in Health, New Zealand 1999, released in 2000,[24] and Reducing Inequalities in Health, released in 2002.[23,24] The former publication firmly put health inequalities on the agenda of the health sector in an authoritative manner as the new Labour Government was beginning to act on these disparities, while the latter publication provided a framework for action to reduce inequalities (Figure 1). The publication provided an entry point for action for health providers who had previously not seen disparities as something they could (or should) act upon, but also clearly demonstrated that action to reduce health disparities could not be implemented by health agencies acting alone, reinforcing the importance of social determinants.

The Ministry of Health, in partnership with an academic institution, the Wellington School of Medicine, undertook the New Zealand Census-Mortality Study, research that directly links census to mortality (and more recently, cancer registration) records. This collaboration led to the publication of four volumes entitled Decades of Disparity, which exhaustively described health inequalities in New Zealand from 1981 to 2004. The reports provide further evidence of the large disparities between Māori and non-Māori, conclusively showing that these disparities were partially independent of socio-economic status.[2,4,14,25] These findings have been crucial in motivating the health sector to act on inequalities. Further research from many other institutions and individuals has illuminated disparities not only in health status, but also in all aspects of the treatment pathway. In addition, the partnership with the university produced the Health Equity Assessment Tool to assist the health sector to plan programmes with due attention to health inequalities (Annex 1). The tool consists of a series of questions that guide planners and providers to consider the drivers of inequalities and how a new or existing programme might impact on the inequalities.[26]

Health strategies developed at both national (Ministry) and local (District Health Board) levels since 2000 have reflected the new commitment to reducing health inequalities. In particular, the overarching New Zealand Health Strategy and New Zealand Disability Strategy, the Māori health strategy He Korowai Oranga, the Primary Health Care Strategy, the Pacific Health and Disability Action Plan, and the Healthy Eating, Healthy Action physical activity and nutrition strategy have provided major impetus to progress on inequalities, clearly identifying inequalities as a priority for both monitoring and action.[27-31] The wide consultation process undertaken in developing these strategies has been an important opportunity to increase awareness in the sector about advances in knowledge on health inequalities and ways to address them. This increased commitment to reducing inequalities is now also seen in the plans of District Health Board plans and, more slowly, in those of the new Primary Health Organizations.

Health inequalities have also become a key focus of health monitoring with an explicit mandate to monitor disparities in the plans of District Health Boards and Primary Health Organizations. The inclusion of the questions on racial discrimination in the New Zealand Health survey has allowed subsequent ground-breaking analyses on the relationship of racial discrimination to health status and new insights into the contribution of discrimination to health inequalities.[8,32]

The past decade has thus seen a reorientation of the New Zealand health sector at the policy level to take action on health inequalities, driven by public and political concern and supported by research evidence. A range of programmes has been undertaken involving many sectors. By way of illustration, an innovation involving the primary health care sector and multi-sectoral collaboration between the housing and health sectors is described in the next section.

6. Primary health care: strategy and implementation

6.1 The problem

Several attempts have been made to reform primary health care in New Zealand since the beginning of the 20th century.[33,34] These reforms had been unsuccessful in shifting the model of care from doctor-owned and -controlled general practices, which maintained the right to set patient charges and resulted in a mismatch between patient need and service availability and access. Inequitable access at this first level of care had a system-wide effect as the general practices acted as gatekeepers for access to the wider health system.

Figure 1: Reducing inequalities in health framework

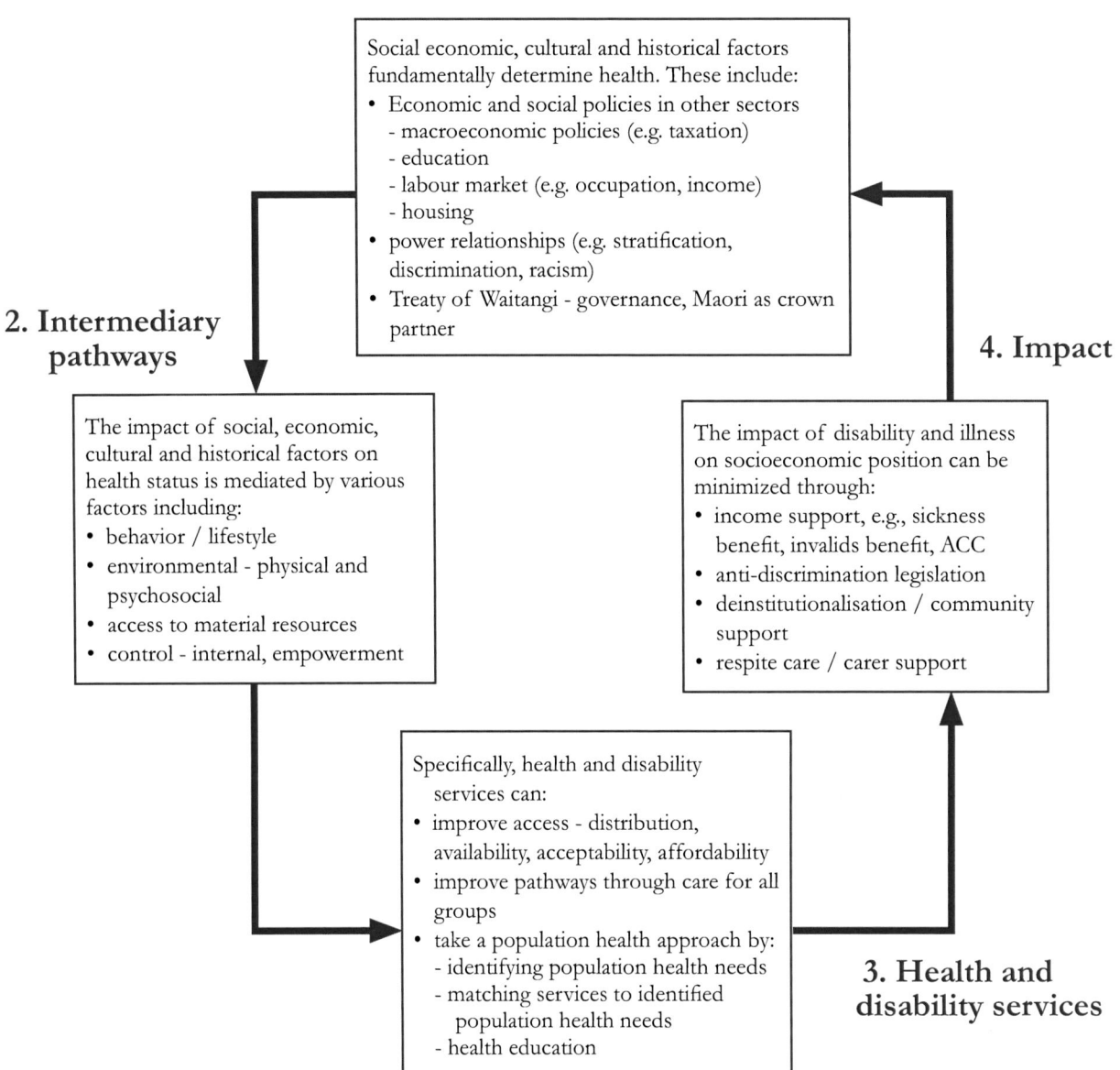

6.2 The evidence

The existing system and its limitations were thoroughly examined. The findings were summarized in a review,[35] which also looked at local and international evidence. A number of barriers to access to effective primary health care were identified, such as: fee-for-service payments, funding not being allotted according to need, co-payments discouraging access by high-need groups, ineffective services for some populations, and lack of services for those most likely to benefit.

6.3 Policy process

A major boost to the development of primary health care in New Zealand came with the launch of the Primary Health Care Strategy[36] in February 2001 and its subsequent implementation. The Strategy was seen as a way to tackle health inequalities from the outset. It provides a clear direction for the development of primary health care and states that a new vision will be achieved over a five- to ten-year period, where:

> People will be part of local primary health care services that improve their health, keep them well, are easy to get to and coordinate their ongoing care. Primary health care services will focus on better health for the population, and **actively work to reduce health inequalities between different groups**.[36]

The Strategy places greater emphasis on population health and recognises the role of the community and preventive care. It views primary health care as involving a range of professionals in service delivery and recognizes the advantages of funding based on population needs rather than fees for service.

The Strategy has the following six key directions:
- to work with local communities and enrolled populations;
- to identify and remove health inequalities;
- to offer access to comprehensive services to improve, maintain and restore people's health;
- to coordinate care across service areas;
- to develop the primary health care workforce; and
- to continuously improve quality using good information.

6.4 Implementation process

This Strategy was implemented through new organizations known as Primary Health Organisations (PHOs). Six years on, PHOs have enrolled 95% percent of the total population and the District Health Boards can now directly influence access barriers such as fees, availability and service design.

PHOs are funded by the Government through District Health Boards to provide a set of essential primary health care services to the enrolled population. At a minimum, this includes services directed towards improving and maintaining the health of the population, as well as providing first-level care. PHOs are expected to involve their communities in their governing processes and all providers and practitioners in their decision-making, rather than one group being dominant. They are not-for-profit bodies and are required to be fully and openly accountable for all public funds that they receive. PHOs receive extra funding to improve access for Māori, Pacific and low-income populations through the development of outreach and other services.

The funding of PHOs does not fully remove the co-payment made by patients. More public funding is offered to areas with the most deprived communities, with a requirement that fees are eliminated for children and are set below an agreed low level for adults.

6.5 Results

Evidence from the formative evaluation[37] and the experience from the community-led services[38] suggest that this model will improve both access and the range of services available. Evidence of improved access for high need groups has been documented.[39] The way people think about health is also changing, as seen in the following quote from a community representative on a PHO:

> We are endeavoring to [influence] the determinants of health. So we have been putting a lot of work into housing, poor housing, youth, employment, recreational facilities, lifestyle, the district council. If you had to say what the difference is between us and the IPA, which looked after the clinical side, we've moved a lot into the actual... determinants. [37]

An example of how health and housing sectors are working together is given in the sections below.

7. Healthy housing programme: public health, public housing, joint action

7.1 The problem

The main catalyst for the Healthy Housing Programme was a group B meningococcal epidemic in New Zealand which began in 1991 and resulted in levels of meningococcal disease approximately ten times higher than those in other developed countries. Further, ethnic disparities were observed in the incidence of the disease with extremely high rates of infection in young (under five years-old) Māori and Pacific children in South Auckland.[40]

7.2 The evidence

A case-control study showed that, overcrowding was the most important risk factor during the epidemic, with an odds ratio of 10.8 for each extra person per room in a home (compared with odds ratios of less than two for other environmental factors, such as tobacco smoke).[41] These findings led to the Healthy Housing Programme and the subsequent development and rollout of an epidemic strain-specific vaccine. The Chief Executive Officer of Housing New Zealand (HNZ), the main provider of social housing, was a powerful advocate for the Healthy Housing Programme, voicing the aim that "no child should die because of the state of their house."[42]

7.3 The policy process

The strategic policy orientation of the health sector towards inequalities and intersectoral action has been described above.

7.4 Implementation

The Healthy Housing Programme was initiated in Auckland in December 2000 as an 18-month pilot. Housing New Zealand Corporation is a Crown agency that manages housing worth more than $11 billion, including 66,000 state houses. The programme was a collaboration between this agency and health agencies in the Auckland region (Auckland Health, now Counties Manukau District Health Board, and the regional public health services provider for the region, Auckland Regional Public Health Service).

In this initiative, the government agencies consulted with community organizations, including NGOs, churches and local governments active in the area. The concern about meningococcal disease was widely shared by government agencies and community alike.

Following consultation, a programme was developed that provided a joint housing and health intervention, capitalizing on the strengths of the three organizations involved. The three aims of the programme agreed upon by the partners were: to reduce crowding levels in HNZ properties; to reduce the risk of meningococcal disease; and to implement intersectoral measures that reduce housing-related disease.

Locations for the programme were chosen by reviewing the avoidable hospitalization rates associated with crowding-related infectious disease, along with measures of poverty and general overcrowding rates. Individual houses within the locations were chosen in the pilot according to high risk for crowding from HNZ tenant data, but as the programme progressed, all HNZ properties in the target locations were assessed.

The initial intervention consisted of a visit by a HNZ official and a public health nurse to assess the needs of the tenants. A joint assessment tool was used whereby the housing official discussed the housing needs of the family and inspected the house while the public health nurse undertook a comprehensive health assessment of all household members and aimed to increase access to primary health services and knowledge of health promoting practices. Baseline data collected included information on avoidable hospitalizations, level of crowding (using a crowding ratio) and a meningococcal disease risk ratio, to help to prioritize families for housing improvements.

Following this, the HNZ official assessed the housing improvements needed and implemented these. These improvements included simple maintenance, ventilation and insulation improvements, transfers to larger accommodation, and extensions to the existing property. The New Zealand Institute of Architects was consulted to assist with the design of the improvements to maximize the health benefit.

Meanwhile, the public health nurse arranged any necessary referrals to health service providers. The nurses involved were very experienced and, as such, were able to contribute a range of practical assistance beyond the health sector. Referrals were thus also made to other social service agencies.

7.5 The results

Almost 5,000 families have had a combined health and housing intervention (mainly capital investment), at a cost of NZ$ 60 million (US$ 45.4 million) aimed at improving access to health services and reducing risks to health from the housing environment. This has resulted in improved health of HNZ tenants, reduced crowding, and improvements to the housing stock. Housing-related avoidable hospitalizations were reduced by 37% in programme homes, compared to a control group. A cost-benefit analysis suggested a positive benefit-to-cost ratio of 1.15 for HNZ. In other words, the programme resulted in a net financial gain when housing benefits and hospital admissions were considered, without taking into account the economic value of reduced admissions, and other non-quantifiable social benefits such as the reported increased wellbeing and community participation among HNZ tenants. The programme is one example of intersectoral action to address health inequalities, since 50% of participants are Pacific families and 25% are Māori families.[43]

The Healthy Housing Programme has encouraged intersectoral collaboration between the health and housing sectors in other parts of the country, particularly with regard to insulation schemes. The spread of this concept has been greatly aided by the realization that benefits accrue over a short period (months, not decades) to both the Health and Housing agencies (good return on investment for housing and reduced admissions for health) as well as providing benefits for communities.

It should be noted that this programme was not the only response to the meningococcal epidemic. During this time, the Government developed a vaccine and delivered it to people below 20 years of age, with an initial focus on the South Auckland community, where rates of the disease were highest. In effect, interventions occurred at all levels, reducing social stratification, diminishing specific exposures, decreasing vulnerability, and improving health service provision.

8. Impact of changing health policy on health inequalities

Although the story of New Zealand's focus on health inequalities is still incomplete, there is emerging data which suggests that ethnic inequalities in health are decreasing and inequalities according to socio-economic status are stabilizing. Figure 2 shows that the life expectancy gap between Māori and non-Māori narrowed from the 1950s through the 70s, widened during the 1980s and 90s, and may now be narrowing once more.[25] Figure 3 shows trends in absolute and relative inequality in all-cause mortality over the period 1981 to 2004, with ages (1–74 years) and sexes pooled.

The apparent turning point in health inequality between 1996 to 1999 and 2001 to 2004 is of great interest. The pattern is at least consistent with the widening of health inequalities occurring after a very short lag following the increase in social inequality caused by the structural reforms begun in 1984. The observed turnaround coincides (after a similarly short lag) with the changes in government policy described above in the health sector and also in the broader social sectors, including increased regulation of the labour and housing markets and increased social assistance. However, it also coincides with improved performance of the New Zealand economy, with greatly reduced unemployment rates. As such, it is difficult to attribute the improvement in health inequality to either one of these factors exclusively—both are likely to have contributed to the recent narrowing in both socio-economic and ethnic inequalities in health.

Figure 2: Life expectancy at birth, by ethnic group and sex, 1950-1952 to 2000-2002

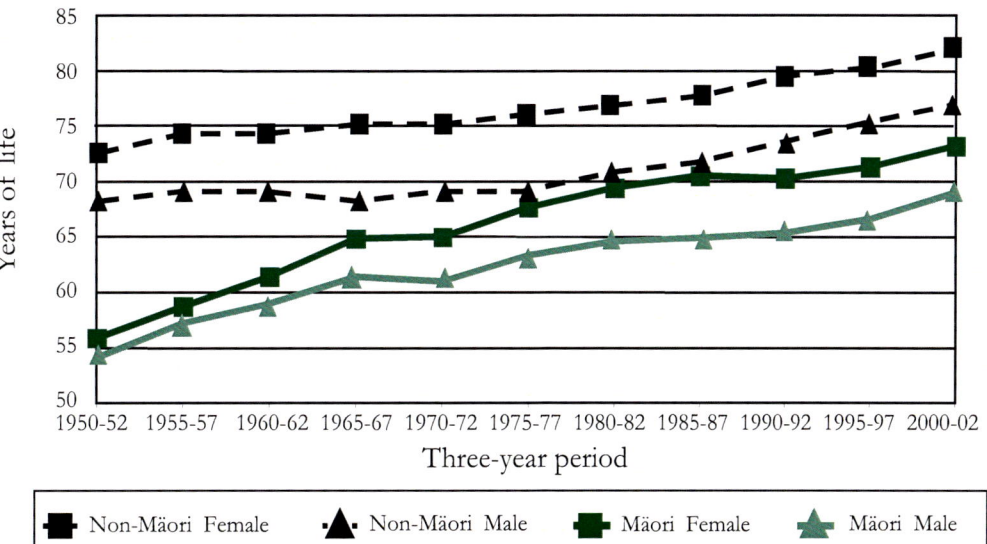

Figure 3: Changes in health inequalities in New Zealand 1981-2004

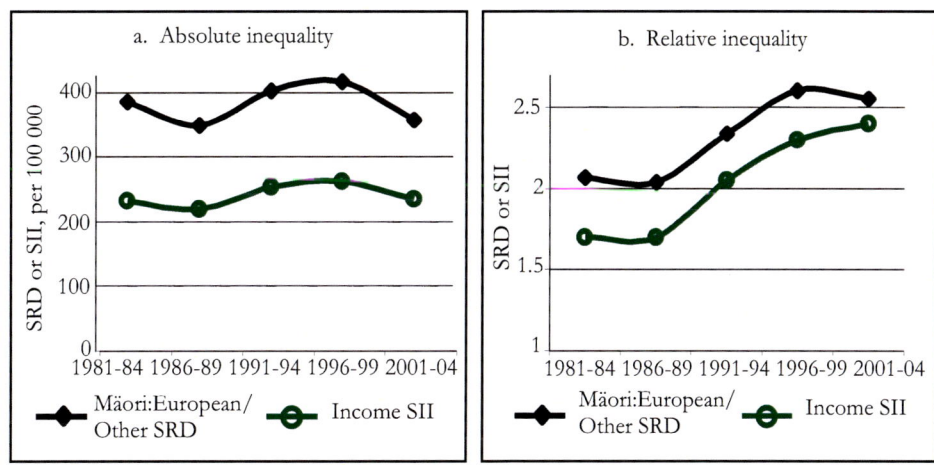

SRD: standardized rate difference (SRD) for Māori compared to European/Other ethnic group (i.e., non-Māori, non-Pacific, non-Asian)
SRR: standardized rate ratio (SRR) for Māori compared to European/Other ethnic groups (i.e. non-Māori, non-Pacific, non-Asian)
SII: slope index of inequality by equivalised household income[3]
RII: relative index of inequality by equivalised household income[4]

---

3 SII and RII are regression-based equivalents of the SRD and SRR.
4 Standardization is to the WHO World Population. Incomes are adjusted for CPI movements and equalized for household size and composition.

9. Conclusion

This paper describes New Zealand's experience in reorienting its health and social policy to prioritize the goal of reducing health inequalities. Much has been achieved in a very short period. The planning of health interventions and the monitoring of their effects are now strongly informed by the need to consider health disparities. However, as has been discussed in this paper, this is very much an incomplete narrative. Despite the impressive changes in policy and strategies, implementation remains variable, even given the existence of innovative projects and approaches such as the Healthy Housing Programme and the Primary Healthcare Strategy described above.

Evidence suggests that the overall change in policy direction has contributed to a reduction in health inequalities in New Zealand. The evidence, however, is inconclusive. In many ways this reflects one of the major difficulties for social policy that aims to address the social determinants of health—the effects are long-term over multiple programme areas, yet the perceived costs of any such policy are immediate.

Sustaining the will to continue with such programmes remains an ongoing challenge for the Ministry of Health and the health sector. In New Zealand, the prioritization of action on health inequalities for Māori was the subject of strong criticism in 2004,[44] which directly resulted in a review of these programmes by the Government. However, the impressive body of evidence accumulated to document health inequalities has assisted in maintaining the consistency of health policy in relation to disparities. It is important to note that the Government has played a central role in facilitating research evidence and moving evidence-based policy development forward, in concert with academia and civil society. New Zealand's experience with this is different from many other countries and this broad consensus improves the chances of sustaining action to address health inequalities over the long term.

With continued policy attention and robust evaluation to demonstrate that policies aimed at reducing health inequality are having the desired effect, New Zealand has a chance of substantially reducing inequalities over the decade.

References

Acheson D. 1998. *Independent Inquiry into Inequalities in Health*. London: The Stationery Office.
Howden-Chapman P, Tobias M (eds). 2000. *Social Inequalities in Health: New Zealand 1999*. Wellington: Ministry of Health.
Minister of Health. 2000. *The New Zealand Health Strategy*. Wellington: Ministry of Health.
Ministry of Health, Public Health Consultancy, Te Roopu Rasngahau Hauora a Eru Pomare. 2002. A Health Equity Assessment Tool. Department of Public Health, University Otago and Ministry of Health
Woodward A, Kawachi I. 2000. Why reduce health inequalities? *Journal of Epidemiology and Community Health* 54(12):923.

Endnotes[5]

1. Whitehead, M. A typology of actions to tackle social inequalities in health. *Journal of Epidemiology & Community Health*. 2007, 61: 473-8.
2. Ministry of Health. *Decades of disparity I. Ethnic mortality trends in New Zealand 1989-1999*. Ministry of Health and University of Otago, Editors. Ministry of Health, Wellington, 2003.
3. Ministry of Health. *Tatau kahukura. Māori health chart book*. Ministry of Health, Wellington, 2006.
4. Ministry of Health. *Decades of disparity III. Ethnic and socio-economic inequalities in mortality, New Zealand 1981-1999*. Ministry of Health, Wellington, 2006.
5. Pearce, N.E. *et al.* Mortality and social class in New Zealand III: male mortality by ethnic group. New Zealand Medical Journal, 1984, 97:31-5.
6. Sporle, A., N. Pearce, and P. Davis, *Social class mortality differences in Maori and non-Maori men aged 15-64 during the last two decades*. New Zealand Medical Journal, 2002. 115: p. 127-31.
7. Ministry of Health. *Tobacco Trends 2006*. Ministry of Health, Wellington, 2007.
8. Harris, R. *et al.* Effects of self-reported racial discrimination and deprivation on Mori health and inequalities in New Zealand: cross-sectional study. *Lancet*, 2006, 367: 2005-09.
9. Davis, P. *et al.* Quality of hospital care for Maori patients in New Zealand: retrospective cross-sectional assessment. *Lancet*, 2006, 367:1920-5.
10. Ministry of Health. *Tupu ola moui. Pacific health chart book 2004*. Ministry of Health, Wellington, 2004
11. Rasanathan, K., D. Craig, and R. Perkins. The novel use of "Asian" as an ethnic category in the New Zealand health sector. *Ethnicity & Health*, 2006, 11:211-27.
12. McDonald, J.T. and S. Kennedy. Insights into the 'healthy immigrant effect': health status and health service use of immigrants to Canada. *Social Science & Medicine*, 2004, 59:1613-27.
13. Ministry of Health. *Asian health chart book*. Ministry of Health, Wellington, 2006.
14. Ministry of Health and University of Otago. *Decades of disparity II. Socio-economic mortality trends in New Zealand 1981-99*. Ministry of Health, Wellington, 2005.
15. Tobias, M. and L.C. Yeh. Do all ethnic groups in New Zealand exhibit socio-economic mortality gradients? *Australian & New Zealand Journal of Public Health*, 2006, 30:343-9.
16. Pearce, J. and D. Dorling. Increasing geographical inequalities in health in New Zealand, 1980-2001. *International Journal of Epidemiology*, 2006, 35:597-603.
17. Te Roopu Rangahau Hauora a Eru Pomare. *Hauora: Maori standards of health III*. Wellington School of Medicine, University of Otago, Wellington, 1995.
18. Reid, P., B. Robson, and R. Jones. Disparities in health: common myths and uncommon truths. *Pacific Health Dialog*, 2000, 7:38-48.
19. Durie, M. *Whaiora: Maori health development*. 2nd ed. Oxford University Press, Auckland, 1998.
20. National Advisory Committee on Health and Disability. *The social, cultural and economic determinants of health in New Zealand*. National Advisory Committee on Health and Disability, Wellington, 1998.
21. Salmond, C. and P. Crampton. NZDep96 - what does it measure? *Social Policy Journal of New Zealand*, 2001, 17:82-100.
22. Clark, H. Budget Address. Parliament, Wellington, 2000.
23. Tobias, M. and P. Howden-Chapman, eds. *Social inequalities in health, New Zealand 1999: a summary*. Ministry of Health, Wellington, 1999.
24. Ministry of Health. *Reducing inequalities in health.*, Ministry of Health, Wellington, 2002.
25. Ministry of Health. *Tracking disparities. Trends in ethnic and socio-economic inequalities in mortality, 1981 - 2004*. Ministry of Health, Wellington, 2007.
26. Ministry of Health, ed. *The Pacific Health and Disability Action Plan*. Ministry of Health, Wellington, 2002.
27. Ministry of Health. *Healthy eating – healthy action. Oranga kai – oranga pumau: a strategic framework*. Ministry of Health, Wellington, 2003.

---

5   All Ministry of Health publications are available from *www.moh.govt.nz/publications*.

28. Ministry of Health. *Primary health care strategy*. Ministry of Health, Wellington, 2001.
29. Ministry of Health. *New Zealand disability strategy*. Ministry of Health, Wellington, 2001.
30. Ministry of Health. *He korowai oranga: Māori health strategy*. Ministry of Health, Wellington, 2001.
31. Ministry of Health. *New Zealand health strategy*. Ministry of Health, Wellington, 2000.
32. Harris, R. *et al.* Racism and health: the relationship between experience of racial discrimination and health in New Zealand. *Social Science & Medicine*, 2006. 63:1428-41.
33. Hay, I. *The caring commodity: the provision of health care in New Zealand*. Oxford University Press, Auckland, 1989.
34. Pool, I. *Te Iwi Maori; A New Zealand Population: Past, Present and Projected*. Auckland University Press, Auckland, 1991.
35. National Health Committee. *Improving Health of New Zealanders by Investing in Primary Health Care*. National Health Committee, Wellington, 2000.
36. Ministry of Health. *The Primary Health Care Strategy*. Ministry of Health, Wellington, 2001.
37. Health Services Research Centre. *Evaluation of the Implementation and Intermediate Outcomes of the Primary Health Care Strategy, First Report: Overview in Evaluation of the Implementation and Intermediate Outcomes of the Primary Health Care Strategy*. Health Services Research Centre, Victoria University, Wellington, 2005.
38. Crampton, P. *et al.* Does community-governed non-profit primary care improve access to services? Cross-sectional survey of practice characteristics. *International Journal of Health Services*, 2005, 35:465-478.
39. Cumming, J. and B. Gribben. *Evaluation of the Primary Health Care Strategy: Practice data analysis 2001-2005*. In *Implementation and intermediate outcomes evaluation of the primary health care strategy*. Health Services Research Centre, Victoria University, Wellington, 2007.
40. O'Hallahan, J. *et al.* From secondary prevention to primary prevention: a unique strategy that gives hope to a country ravaged by meningococcal disease. *Vaccine*, 2005, 23:2197-201.
41. Baker, M. *et al.* Household crowding a major risk factor for epidemic meningococcal disease in Auckland children. *Pediatric Infectious Disease Journal*, 2000, 19:983-90.
42. Matheson, D. Personal communication with CEO Housing NZ. 2003.
43. Bourke, I., *Healthy housing programme evaluation*. Briefing paper to Minister of Health and Minister of Housing (unpublished). 2006.
44. Towns, C. *et al.* The Orewa Speech: another threat to Maori health? *New Zealand Medical Journal*, 2004, 117:U1145.

Annex

A health equity assessment tool (equity lens) for tackling inequalities in health May 2004

There is considerable evidence, both internationally and in New Zealand, of significant inequalities in health between socio-economic groups, ethnic groups, people living in different geographical regions and males and females (Acheson 1998; Howden-Chapman and Tobias 2000).

Research indicates that the poorer you are, the worse your health. In some countries with a colonial history, indigenous people have poorer health than others.

Reducing inequalities is a priority for the Government. The New Zealand Health Strategy acknowledges the need to address health inequalities as 'a major priority requiring ongoing commitment across the sector' (Minister of Health 2000).

Inequalities in health are unfair and unjust. They are also not natural; they are the result of social and economic policy and practices. Therefore, inequalities in health are avoidable (Woodward and Kawachi 2000).

The following set of questions has been developed to assist you to consider how particular inequalities in health have come about, and where the effective intervention points are to tackle them. They should be used in conjunction with the Ministry of Health's Intervention Framework (Ministry of Health 2002).

1. What health issue is the policy/programme trying to address?
2. What inequalities exist in this health area?
3. Who is most advantaged and how?
4. How did the inequality occur? (What are the mechanisms by which this inequality was created, maintained or increased?)
5. What are the determinants of this inequality?
6. How will you address the Treaty of Waitangi in the context of the New Zealand Public Health and Disability Act 2000?
7. Where/how will you intervene to tackle this issue? Use the Ministry of Health Intervention Framework to guide your thinking.
8. How could this intervention affect health inequalities?
9. Who will benefit most?
10. What might the unintended consequences be?
11. What will you do to make sure it does reduce/eliminate inequalities?
12. How will you know if inequalities have been reduced/eliminated?

(Adapted from Bro Taf Authority. 2000. Planning for Positive Impact: Health inequalities impact assessment tool. Cardiff: Bro Taf Authority.)

Amended by Ministry of Health. May 2004.

Source: Te Roopu Rangahau a Erū Pomare., Ministry of Health and Public Health Consultancy. 2003. A Health Equity Assessment Tool. Wellington: Public Health Consultancy, Wellington School of Medicine and Health Sciences.

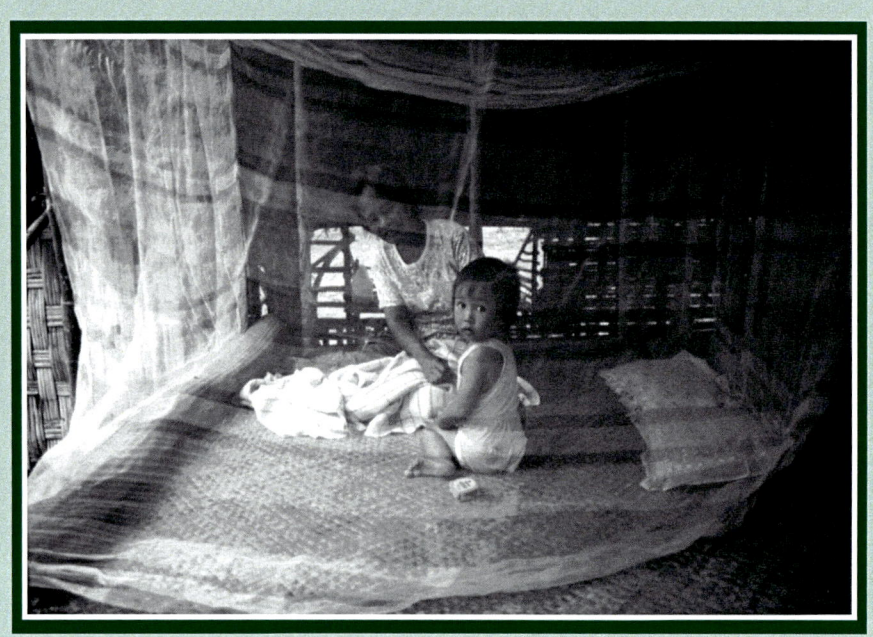

The development and targeting of malaria control interventions for populations in high transmission areas of Cambodia: the influence of research on policy and practice

Sean Hewitt[1]; Roberto Garcia[1]; Nong Sao Kry[2]; Chea Ngoun[2]; Abdur Rashid[3]; Esther Sedano[1]; Kheng Sim[2]; Tho Sochantha[2]; Doung Socheat[2]; Srey Socheath[2]

1. Summary

Based on evidence from the National Malaria Centre's (CNM) bednet intervention study, which started in 2000, a pilot project was established in 2001 to assess the viability of providing village-based diagnosis and treatment for malaria in Cambodia's least accessible and most highly endemic communities. Services were delivered through a network of village-based volunteers equipped with rapid diagnostic tests, heat-stable artesunate suppositories and pre-packaged artemisinin-based combination therapy. This European Commision-supported pilot was a success, and the Village Malaria Worker scheme was adopted by the Ministry of Health as the malaria diagnosis and treatment delivery strategy of choice for remote malaria hot-spots. The project has since scaled-up with support from the Global Fund to fight Tuberculosis, AIDS and Malaria (Global Fund), GTZ and WHO to cover all of Cambodia's 300 inaccessible and highly endemic villages. A similar community-based approach for malaria control in remote transmission hot-spots has been adopted or is under development in Viet Nam, Thailand, Lao People's Democratic Republic, Myanmar and China.

Following on from the surveys carried out for identifying target villages during the expansion of the Village Malaria Worker scheme and to provide a robust baseline for the assessment of Global Fund support, a consortium was commissioned by WHO to carry out a malaria baseline survey in 2004. The survey, implemented by the Institute of Public Health, collected malaria data from a broadly representative sample of communities within 2 kilometres of the forest (with some extended survey data from up to 5 kilometres). Survey results demonstrated the clear decline in the risk of malaria with increasing distance from the forest edge. However, findings indicated that malaria risk was higher immediately adjacent to the forest than had previously been supposed. On the basis of this finding, interventions were re-targeted: the inclusion threshold for free bednet delivery based on forest proximity was raised from 0.2 kilometres to 1 kilometre.

This paper documents the development of the Village Malaria Worker scheme, from the origin of the concept, through to the pilot phase, technical dissemination, political lobbying, formal adoption by Ministry of Health, and, national roll-out. This paper also presents the

---

1 European Commission- Cambodia Malaria Control Project
2 National Malaria Center
3 World Health Organization, Cambodia

development and implementation of the subsequent national malaria baseline survey and reports on how the resulting data were used to improve the targeting of malaria control interventions.

The methodology applied to influence policy and practice is reviewed, its effectiveness assessed and the lessons learned as a result presented.

2. The problem

Even in 2001, Cambodia's malaria control programme was rather advanced and included large-scale use of insecticide-treated bednets (ITN), state-of-the-art rapid diagnostic tests (RDT) and pre-packaged artemisinin-based combination therapy (pACT) as well as an innovative public-private mixed approach to the provision of early diagnosis and appropriate treatment (EDAT). The public sector provided microscopic or RDT-based diagnosis and pACT through a slowly expanding network of health outlets and the Malarine social marketing project provided the same RDTs and pACT (this time with glossy, tamper-proof packaging) through the private sector. Despite this two-pronged approach, an important gap in service provision remained and, paradoxically, it was the very poorest communities in the least accessible and most malaria-prone areas that were left unprotected.

2.1 Purpose

To address this issue and develop a truly comprehensive national strategy, a pilot project was established in 2001 to investigate the viability of providing village-based EDAT for malaria through a network of volunteers equipped with RDTs, heat-stable artesunate suppositories and pACT. Surveys associated with the subsequent scale-up of village-based EDAT revealed the very focal nature of malaria transmission in Cambodia and highlighted the need for a national malariametric survey and an in-depth review of how malaria control interventions were being targeted by the National Malaria Control Programme.

2.2 Introduction and brief history

Since 2000, Provincial Health Departments in Cambodia have been providing microscopic or RDT-based diagnosis and pre-packaged combination therapy through hospitals, health centres and a slowly expanding network of health posts. In addition, they have been providing referral and emergency care of severe or complicated cases at operational district centres. In theory, anyone within reach of a public health facility can access free health care through this system. In reality, however, it is usually only members of poorer households living near a health facility or people who have tried the private sector without success who seek care in this way.

With increased efforts to reform the health sector, the situation is now improving. However, it will take time to build people's faith in the public sector. Recent surveys revealed that 80% of malaria sufferers choose private sector health facilities in preference to public.[2]

The private sector is vast and unregulated. Recent undercover surveys in Phnom Penh revealed that 49% of consultations with private medical practitioners resulted in the prescription of potentially hazardous treatments.[3] The situation outside the major urban centres is likely to be even worse, as most private healthcare in Cambodia is provided not by doctors, but by the *nhek luok thnam* (village drug sellers). Most have little or no training, so inappropriate prescription of a cocktail of drugs is the norm. Often the quality of drugs is substandard and, despite recent efforts by the Ministry of Health, fake drugs remain a problem in some outlets. Pharmaceutical anarchy is one of the most formidable obstacles to rational reform of the health sector in Cambodia.

In an effort to address these problems, the Ministry for Health adopted an innovative social marketing approach to provide access to appropriate, low-cost early diagnosis and treatment for falciparum malaria through the private sector. This has become known as the Malarine Project and is now managed by PSI and funded by the Global Fund. In addition to providing RDTs and pACT, the project educates high-risk groups about the importance of proper diagnosis and compliance with recommended regimens. Success relies to a great extent on the educational status of the target audience because, although the products are subsidized, they are not cheap when compared with the alternatives offered by the *nhek luok thnam* (where 'clinical' diagnosis is free and a single tablet of dihydroartemisinin, which may give temporary relief, costs just US$ 0.2).

Not surprisingly, the Malarine Project is proving most effective where the population is relatively well-educated and has access to advertising, cash and private sector outlets. Provinces with such a population include Battambang and Pursat, which together have most of the multi-drug resistant falciparum malaria in Cambodia. It is hoped that, in time, the Malarine Project will have a profound and lasting impact on the drug resistance profile of parasites in this region, reversing the currently rising trends. Withdrawal of monotherapies from the market and introduction of the Global ACT Subsidy, which will reduce the price of approved ACTs in the private sector to roughly the same price as chloroquine, will help a lot in this regard.

The public-private mixed approach for malaria control described above left a very important gap: a section of the community that was beyond the reach of both public sector health facilities and the Malarine Project. The group that was neglected was made up of the very poorest communities in the least accessible areas, but it is these communities that bear the greatest malaria burden.

Surveys conducted by the CNM in Ratanakiri in September 2001 revealed a mean falciparum prevalence in children under fifteen of 41% (ranging from 7% on the outskirts of the provincial capital to 81% in the periphery). It was estimated from these surveys that hyperendemic malaria persists in more than 50% of villages in this northeastern province.

Although in areas of intense transmission immunity does develop with time, malaria-related morbidity and mortality among children are very high. Malaria during pregnancy commonly results in severe maternal anaemia and vulnerable low birth weight children (especially in primigravidae).

Extrapolating from studies conducted in Africa, the CNM made a tentative estimate that almost 20% of the deaths among children under the age of five in hyperendemic areas of Cambodia may have been directly due to malaria and another 20% may have had malaria as a major contributory factor. At the time, an estimated 100,000 Cambodians were living in remote hyperendemic malaria hot-spots beyond reasonable reach of conventional health care.

Nationwide demographic and health surveys conducted in 2000 estimated under-five mortality in Cambodia at 121.6 per thousand. For Ratanakiri province, this figure rose to 229.3 per thousand.[5] However, the over-dispersed distribution of health problems in general and the very focal nature of malaria in particular meant that the situation might have been considerably worse in the least accessible villages. Anecdotal reports suggested that under-five mortality might have exceeded 400 per thousand in the worst affected communities.

2.3 Prevailing political climate

During the Khmer Rouge period (1975 to 1979) the National Malaria Control Programme collapsed completely and during the long aftermath its recovery was slow. Since the late 1990s, however, with support from WHO and other donors, growth in the capacity of the CNM has been dramatic. By 2001, the CNM was developing one of the most up-to-date and effective national malaria control programmes in the world. The CNM had four senior malaria advisers (two from WHO, one from the European Commission and one from World Bank/Department for International Development [DfID] funding) and a growing number of national staff returning from overseas with relevant postgraduate training. In addition, a number of NGOs, including Partners for Development, Health Unlimited, Nomad, Malteser and Médecins Sans Frontières (MSF) were taking an active part in malaria control at district level in selected provinces. The malaria situation was still serious, but there was a spirit of innovation and the National Malaria Control Programme was growing steadily, with strong support from the Ministry of Health.

3. Development of strategy and evidence

In 2001, the CNM (supported by EC) initiated a large village-scale study of bednet efficacy in Ratanakiri in the northeast of the country.[6] In order to provide essential health cover for all of the villagers in the bednet study group, a network of volunteers was established to provide EDAT. Following on from the early success of the strategy in these study communities, CNM piloted village-based EDAT as an intervention in its own right in 36 ethnic minority communities in the northeast of the country and in ten Khmer communities in Koh Kong province in the southwest.

In agreement with community leaders, one person from each of the 46 target villages was selected to be a Village Malaria Worker. Each Worker was taught how to recognize the symptoms of malaria, reduce a fever, use the Paracheck F® test, treat where indicated, and refer patients as necessary to the nearest health facility. In addition, they were taught how to keep simple written records of all tests conducted (detailing results and treatments given) and of any deaths occurring in the village.

Despite the very low level of education of many of the Village Malaria Workers, regular monitoring visits (bi-weekly initially and then monthly) and routine feedback indicated that, in the vast majority of cases, they worked well. In the first ten months of implementation in Ratanakiri 4,804 patients presented to Village Malaria Workers (from a study population of approximately 11,000) and 2,271 of these tested positive for falciparum malaria and were treated. In Koh Kong, 714 patients from a population of 2,200 presented and 254 tested positive and were treated.

Prior to launch, many health workers believed that suppositories would not be acceptable therapies in ethnic minority and rural Khmer communities, but the use of Plasmotrim® suppositories has been remarkably well accepted. Of the 1,099 RDT positive children under the age of six seen in Ratanakiri during the first ten months, 1,059 were given a five-day course of Plasmotrim® (in addition to mefloquine). In each case, the Village Malaria Worker demonstrated the application of the first dose to patient's parent/guardian. The remaining doses were not generally supervised, but feedback suggests that compliance was high. Fewer than 5% of parents formally rejected the use of suppositories (these individuals were given ground artesunate tablets instead). Suppositories were also well received by all 23 falciparum-positive children detected during the first four months of the Koh Kong pilot study. Again feedback suggests that compliance with the full regimen was high.

A sociological study conducted by Brown *et al.* (2002) as part of the pilot assessment process in four Ratanakiri communities revealed considerable differences in treatment-seeking behaviour between villages with and without Village Malaria Workers. In villages with Village Malaria Workers, 70% of children under five received treatment within three days of onset of febrile illness. This figure fell to 30% in villages without Workers. In addition, where Village Malaria Workers were present, only 10% of under-fives did not get treatment at all, compared with 30% in non-Village Malaria Worker communities. Although only a small number of villages were sampled in this study, these findings were considered indicative, since they were broadly corroborated by informal feedback from other communities covered by the Village Malaria Worker network. The study also indicated that both the availability of Village Malaria Workers and their use by women might be improved if a two-person, mixed-sex team were trained in each target community.

During the first year of the study, 164 deaths were recorded in the 36 Ratanakiri villages. Autopsy interviews are notoriously unreliable, but efforts were made to identify the possible causes of these deaths, based on the symptoms recorded during postmortem interviews with relatives. Of the 122 deaths for which detailed records were available, nine gave positive RDTs. These confirmed malaria deaths at ages less than 1, 1, 2, 2, 4, 8, 12, 35 and 65 years. Six more people were not tested, but were considered probable malaria deaths on the basis of symptoms described. Twelve more died as a result of accidents. Based on reported symptoms, the remaining 95 were considered unlikely to have had malaria at the time of death. Forty-one of these 95 were children under six years and among this group, 18 had coughs, 14 had diarrhoea, five had malaria-like symptoms but negative dipsticks, one had paralysis, two had stomach ache and one had bleeding prior to death.

An estimated under-five mortality rate of 170 per thousand in communities served by Village Malaria Workers compares favourably with the under-five mortality estimates for rural Ratanakiri as a whole (229+ per thousand). Although this estimate is based on a number of extrapolations, it was considered sufficiently robust to demonstrate considerably reduced under-five mortality in the pilot communities.

At the time of the pilot, the annual per capita budget for village-based EDAT was estimated at US$ 1.50 (24% for diagnostic tests and 44% for drugs). Although this per capita cost is high, the intervention was considered cost-effective and the relatively small number of communities in hyperendemic areas meant that the overall cost of scale-up would be low (about US$ 150,000 per annum).

Expansion of the scope of the Village Malaria Worker programme to cover other important health problems, including acute respiratory tract infections and diarrhoea, would greatly improve the cost effectiveness of the scheme and should have an additional major beneficial impact on childhood survival. A pilot study to investigate the feasibility of this approach was initiated by CNM/WHO shortly after the Village Malaria Worker pilot was completed.

A comparison of passive case detection data from Village Malaria Workers in 36 villages[4] with that from rural public sector health facilities revealed that the Village Malaria Worker strategy is particularly effective at targeting children under five years (Figure 1) and it is this group that is at highest risk of death in these hyperendemic and holoendemic[5] communities.

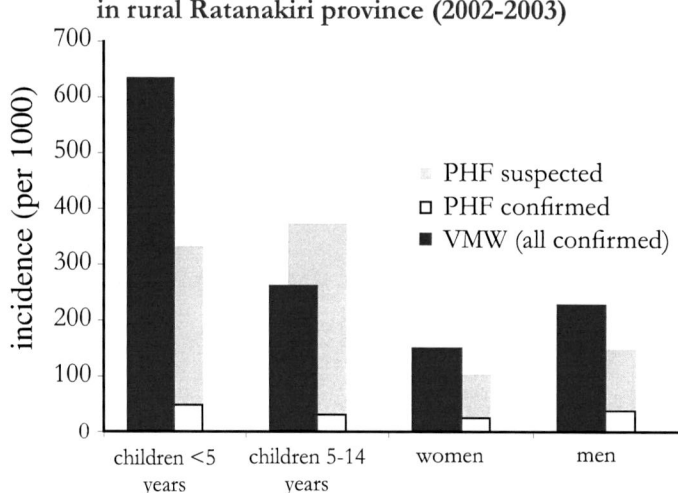

Figure 1. Comparisons of estimates of malaria incidence in rural Ratanakiri province (2002-2003)

The body of evidence described above clearly demonstrated the added value associated with village-based EDAT and provided a solid platform for lobbying for policy change and for funding for scale-up.

3.1 The lobby for expansion

The push for the expansion of village-based EDAT was led by the National Malaria Control Programme, with strong support from the European Commission and WHO. The Ministry of Health had to be convinced that a rather unpalatable change in policy—to allow

---

4 The number of suspected and confirmed cases reported at the PHF are grossly exaggerated (probably in the region of double the real figures). Nevertheless the trends by age group remain real and the effectiveness of Village Malaria Workers reaching children under 5 years old is clear.

5 Endemicity is graded according to the proportion of children aged 2 to 9 years with enlarged spleens: Mesoendemic - low to medium intensity transmission - enlarged spleen rate of 11 to 50%; Hyperendemic - medium to high intensity transmission - enlarged spleen rate of 51 to 75%; and Holoendemic – very high intensity transmission - enlarged spleen rate of greater than 75%.

volunteers with minimal training to administer diagnostic tests and provide treatment—was warranted, given the dire health-related circumstances in highly endemic and inaccessible communities. In order to make the policy change more acceptable, the village-based EDAT approach was proposed as an emergency measure, to be withdrawn following the expansion of health services.

The lobbying process took place at several levels and progress reports from the pilot study were presented to key stakeholders during regular routine weekly meetings at the CNM. A number of newspaper articles were published as the effectiveness of the approach became apparent. Several field visits to remote communities were organized by CNM and the European Commission for senior officials from the Ministry of Health and WHO and for the team conducting the mid-term evaluation of Roll Back Malaria to see village-based EDAT operations for themselves. Preliminary results from the pilot study were presented during these field visits. Senior officials of the Ministry of Health were then kept updated of pilot project progress during informal discussions at a variety of official gatherings.

Final results were presented to a broad-range of stakeholders, including senior officials from the Ministry of Health, during a specially arranged high-profile dissemination event in Phnom Penh. During this meeting the principle of village-based EDAT for communities beyond the reach of conventional health services was formally adopted by the Ministry of Health.

3.2 Implementation of scale-up

Following the success of the Village Malaria Worker pilot project and the adoption of the scheme by the Ministry of Health as the EDAT delivery strategy of choice for remote malaria hot-spots, an application for funding for expansion of the scheme to cover Cambodia's 300 communities most at risk was submitted to the Global Fund Round 2. When the European Commission-Cambodia Malaria Control Programme, which had funded the pilot project, ended in December 2002 WHO and GTZ provided bridging funds to maintain services in the pilot areas while long-term funding was being sought. Once the Global Fund Round 4 application was approved, the GTZ 'Global Fund back-up initiative' provided technical assistance and financial support for the scaling-up process.

An interim Village Malaria Worker project management team was established, pending Global Fund disbursement, and terms of reference for a permanent team were prepared. A detailed protocol was developed for village selection in order to ensure rational targeting of limited resources. The protocol was thoroughly field-tested with the selection teams to ensure that all of the team members adopted a scientifically rigorous approach to the screening process. Robust data collection forms were designed and a data compilation mechanism was set-up.

Preliminary selection of villages was based on proximity to forest as recorded in the national geographic information system (GIS) and was cross-referenced with information from review of detailed maps. Discrepancies between records of forest proximity recorded in the GIS and actual forest proximity were immediately apparent and corrected. This preliminary selection was fine-tuned based on feedback from meetings with health workers at provincial, district and commune level. In the first year of operations, 333 villages were surveyed. In each village, 20 children aged two to nine years were screened for malaria with RDTs and checked for splenomegaly.

As well as being essential for the Village Malaria Worker village selection process, the data generated confirmed that using forest proximity data was likely to be a very effective means of targeting bednets and other malaria control interventions. The vast majority of holoendemic and hyperendemic villages were inside the forest and the vast majority of mesoendemic villages lay within 200 metres of the forest (Figure 2). However the sample of villages surveyed was carefully selected, based on forest cover and so was not representative of villages in general. It was clear that additional surveys in less forested communities would need to be carried out to categorically confirm this observation.

Figure 2. Endemicity of villages by distance from forest

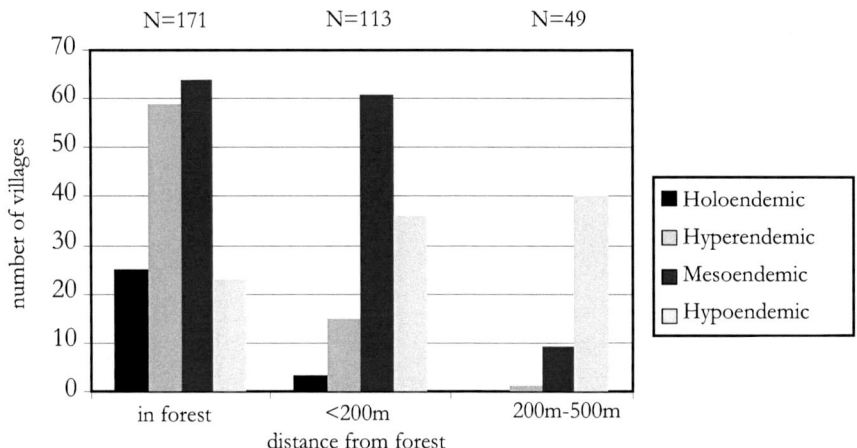

The data collected during the Village Malaria Worker village selection surveys also indicated that the forest cover data from a geographic information system used by CNM for targeting bednet distribution was out of date. The evidence suggested that, in addition to considerable deforestation, there had also been considerable reforestation. While this seems anomalous (and initially raised concerns regarding the validity of the original data), further analysis revealed that the reforestation was largely restricted to three northeastern provinces where rich volcanic soil and relatively high rainfall had combined to result in rapid re-growth of thick, lush vegetation after forest clearance.

It was agreed within CNM that further surveys should be conducted to complete the assessment of the relationship between forest cover and endemicity, and the degree of discrepancy between the GIS-reported figures and actual figures. It was also clear that the classification of ground cover would need to be refined to distinguish between open deciduous woodland (which affords little shade and is therefore not ideal habitat for vector mosquitoes) and dense rainforest, and, similarly, to distinguish between lush humid undergrowth in an area cleared of forest and dry open grassland.

By the end of 2005, rollout of the village-based volunteer network was complete and the 300 most malaria endemic communities in Cambodia were being provided access to EDAT through the Village Malaria Worker project. Rapid roll-out was facilitated greatly by the approach: a vertical CNM-led project, which allowed essential supplies to bypass the delays and other problems inherent in the health network at the time. This emergency-style vertical approach was justified by the atrocious health indicators in the target communities.

3.3 The Cambodia Malaria Baseline Survey (CMBS)

Based on the findings described above and on the need for a robust baseline dataset on which to base future assessments of the programmatic impact of the Global Fund grant, CNM decided to call for a national survey. The CMBS was implemented by the National Institute of Public Health in November/December 2004, under the supervision of a task force which included representatives from all of the key stakeholders involved in malaria control in Cambodia and with technical inputs from the Malaria Consortium and the United States Armed Forces Institute of Medical Science. The CMBS provided baseline data on a broad range of agreed indicators for measuring the progress of the national malaria control programme towards targets set in the Global Fund grant agreements.

The overall slide positivity rate in sampled clusters (which focused on higher risk regions) was 2.7%, rapid diagnostic test positivity rate in nearby clusters was 3.9% and spleen rate 2.9%.[6] As expected, positivity rates were higher nearer to the forest, but there was little difference between distances of 0 to 0.25 kilometres from the forest compared with 0.25 to 1 kilometres from the forest. In contrast, there was a sharp decline in the zone from 1 to 2 kilometres from forest. The key recommendation resulting from the CMBS was that preventive measures should be targeted mainly at populations living up to 1 kilometres from the forest (the strategy at the time was to target communities only up to 0.2 kilometres from the forest).

Other recommendations and observations of the CMBS included:

1. The National Malaria Control Programme could achieve the most impact for its resources by treating and retreating existing nets. The great majority of interviewees were already sleeping under a net, but these were not treated: 48% of children were sleeping under a net that had never been treated, and another 19% were sleeping under nets for which previous treatments had expired.
2. Awareness of how malaria is transmitted and how this can be prevented was found to be high, but awareness of ITNs was very low, so the value of insecticide on nets should be the main message for health education campaigns.
3. Provision of long-lasting insecticidal nets (LLINs) should be targeted at communities within 1 kilometre of the forest. Access to ITNs should also be facilitated beyond 1 kilometre from forest, particularly with a view to protecting people at occupational risk of malaria.
4. Further geographical analysis is needed to determine the most cost-effective and accurate ways of obtaining rapid estimates of village-level risk. This would explore newly available forest cover datasets.

---

6   As malaria is a highly focal disease in Cambodia, a huge sample size would be required to determine the national average, thus the comparison is not available.

5. Intense efforts are needed to reduce ruptures of antimalarial drug stocks in public sector health facilities.
6. Promotion of Malarine in the private sector needs to be handled carefully to minimize unnecessary use of antimalarials by people currently using non-antimalarials for fever. The most promising approach would be to promote the use of parasitological diagnosis to determine the need for treatment. Strategies for increasing access to reliable diagnosis are needed.
7. The higher prevalence of malaria in pregnant than in non-pregnant women warrants further investigation, as it may reflect poorer utilisation of insecticide-treated nets (as indicated by survey results), pointing to the need for more targeted education.
8. Malaria slide positivity is strongly associated with the poorest parts of the population. Poverty reduction strategies should include malaria control measures.
9. For the most part, the process of undertaking the survey worked well. The full engagement of the multi-agency taskforce was crucial to the success of the survey; although it is costly in staff time, it should be maintained as an essential component of follow-up surveys.

3.4 What health outcomes were achieved?

Village-based EDAT has had a profound impact on mortality in target villages. Recorded malaria-related mortality dropped from 15% during the first year after roll-out to 8% last year (Table 2). Pre-intervention levels for malaria-related mortality were probably considerably higher than 15%.

Last year, Village Malaria Workers working in 300 villages tested 84,917 fever cases and treated 43,437 people who had falciparum malaria (Table 1). This compares with 78,700 malaria cases treated in the public sector. Evidence from the pilot study suggests that only around 10% of these cases would have found their way to the public sector if the village-based EDAT scheme had not been introduced. The majority would have been treated by *nhek luok thnam* and some 30% would not have sought treatment at all. Clearly, the contribution of the Village Malaria Workers is immense.

Although morbidity has certainly been dramatically reduced as a result of early treatment shortening the duration of illness, the intervention appears to have had little effect on transmission (despite the simultaneous introduction of high level coverage with LLINs). This is surprising and should be investigated as a high priority. As part of this investigation, in-depth research into the micro-epidemiology of malaria in forest communities should be carried out to identify exactly where people are becoming infected.

Table 1 Malaria cases reported from VMW villages

Year	Total cases tested	Total cases positive	Total deaths from all causes	Malaria confirmed deaths	Malaria suspected deaths
2004	18 771	11 998 (64%)	218	33 (15%)	54 (25%)
2005	50 885	28 443 (56)	527	29 (6%)	35 (7%)
	84 917	43 437 (51%)	421	34 (8%)	25 (6%)
Total	154 573	83 878	1 166	62	89

The village-based EDAT scheme has been wholly complementary to existing public and private sector initiatives within the National Malaria Control Programme. It is an important initiative, which, if supported appropriately, could have a wide reaching and dramatic impact on the health of people living in many of the world's most disadvantaged communities. The methodology developed in Cambodia is broadly applicable to remote highly malaria endemic communities around the world.

The feasibility of introducing oral rehydration salts and cotrimoxazole as add-on interventions for treating diarrhoea and acute respiratory tract infections is being assessed by the Ministry of Health and WHO in a specially designed study. A village-based control strategy addressing the three main killer diseases of children could have major implications both in Cambodia and in the rest of the developing world.

Village-based health care providers are likely to evolve into a new private sector. Already, Village Malaria Workers in some communities have started selling a range of products in an effort to provide for patients presenting with symptoms that are not associated with malaria or for those with malaria symptoms that are RDT negative. It is better that the public sector embraces this enterprise by supporting add-on interventions, than allowing the continued growth of an unregulated and untrained private sector. The introduction of a single nominal charge for consultation payable to the Village Malaria Worker —irrespective of either symptoms or treatment—warrants evaluation, in conjunction with the feasibility study for add-on interventions. Such an incentive scheme would likely further enhance Village Malaria Worker performance.

The CNM's village-based EDAT project is one of the most advanced and mature of its kind. An in-depth review of progress so far should be carried out and the findings should be properly documented in the international literature.

With five similar but unlinked programmes going to scale in Southeast Asia at present, there is clearly a need for an inter-country forum to share experiences. WHO would be well placed to promote such a gathering. A review of the start-up process should be conducted in order to develop a synthesis from the various projects. This would provide a valuable tool for policy development, and facilitate dissemination and advocacy at various levels in order to carry the initiative forward elsewhere. There is now clearly a need for pilot/demonstration projects in West/Central Asia and in Africa.

The CNM and implementing partners involved in the National Malaria Control Programme have made a number of changes in strategy and embarked on a number of new initiatives as a result of the recommendations presented in the CMBS. These include: LLINs, which are now provided for all those living within 1 kilometre of the forest, resulting in the protection of a total of 820,000 people; various initiatives have been introduced to improve access to LLINs for those living outside this zone who are nevertheless at occupational risk of contracting malaria; National Malaria Control Programme is placing greater emphasis on re-treating existing nets, and health education and communication efforts emphasize raising awareness of the value of insecticide on nets. Geographical analysis to determine the most cost-effective and accurate way of obtaining rapid estimates of village-level risk has not yet been initiated, but records of forest proximity have been updated. Efforts to reduce losses of antimalarial drugs from public sector health facilities are ongoing; and PSI is promoting the use of parasitological diagnosis to improve prescription practices linked to Malarine in the private sector.

None of these changes resulting from the CMBS have required high-level approval within the Ministry of Health, as technical management of the National Malaria Control Programme is central to CNM's mandate. Making the changes has therefore been relatively straightforward and is part of the day-to-day running of a dynamic and responsive malaria control programme.

4. Conclusions

The methodology applied to influence the Ministry of Health's policy on EDAT was highly effective. From the early stages of the pilot project, key stakeholders, including political figures and senior staff within the Ministry of Health and within the broader health sector (United Nations agencies, NGOs), were kept informed of progress both at country-level and internationally. Every opportunity was taken to involve influential people in the process and the team evaluating Roll Back Malaria (which included the Executive Director of the Global Fund) visited several communities involved in the Village Malaria Worker pilot project. The lobbying process took place on many different levels and as soon as the likely effectiveness of the intervention became clear, the advocacy was relentless.

It seems likely that the pioneering action of the CNM in the field of village-based EDAT for malaria acted as a trigger for other countries in the region. WHO's involvement in the dissemination process was almost certainly pivotal in this regard. Furthermore, WHO's strong technical support for Global Fund application development in the region has put it in an especially strong position to influence country strategy in a most positive way.

The National Malaria Control Programme was fortunate in that the European Commission-Cambodia Malaria Control Programme provided a very flexible source of funding to support the policy change agenda. The European Commission-Cambodia Malaria Control Programme had also gained considerable experience in the field having been centrally involved with WHO in the development of the Malarine Project.

The adoption of village-based EDAT for malaria by the Ministry of Health resulted in WHO initiating a pilot study to assess the feasibility of developing add-on interventions for the treatment of diarrhoea and acute respiratory tract infections in children. It could certainly be argued that health concerns for people living in remote communities were brought to the fore as a result of village-based EDAT going to scale.

There was no change in the existing structure of health service delivery as a result of this new intervention. Rather, a vertical system was set-up in parallel to the conventional public sector system with its own project management unit within the CNM responsible for training, supply, supervision and monitoring and evaluation. This approach was considered justified given the emergency nature of the intervention. Three years on, this approach should be reviewed in light of improved management and commodity supply at district level.

The adoption of the strategy has had no discernable impact on resource patterns. These were anyway in a state of flux with the closure of the European Commission-Cambodia Malaria Control Programme and the securing of several Global Fund grants for malaria control.

Policy change is probably rather more straightforward in Cambodia than in many other countries in the region. The health sector has evolved rapidly as the political situation has stabilized (following the Khmer Rouge regime and its aftermath), so policy change is not so unusual. Public opinion was not a major influence in the policy change process in this instance.

It is unlikely that a change in policy such as this will have any influence on the ease of future changes at the Ministry of Health end, but at the CNM end, the involvement of senior staff in the process of policy change through the strategic dissemination of research findings will certainly have strengthened capacity in this regard (even though until now, there had been no formal debriefing on the process adopted).

Endnotes

1. Brown, E., *et al. Health beliefs and practices with regards to malaria in ethnic minority communities in Northeast Cambodia.* Unpublished report. Phnom Penh, CNM/European Commission-Cambodia Malaria Control Programme, 2002.
2. Bury, L. *Malaria risk factors study.* Unpublished report. Phnom Penh, CNM/European Commission-Cambodia Malaria Control Programme, 1999.
3. Gollogly, L. The dilemmas of aid: Cambodia 1992-2002. *The Lancet,* 2002, 360:793-798.
4. Hewitt, S. *Technical support to assist the National Malaria Centre in scaling-up village based diagnosis and treatment for malaria in remote hyperendemic hot-spots in Cambodia.* Phnom Penh, Final Report for GTZ, 2004.
5. National Institute of Statistics, Directorate General for Health [Cambodia], and ORC Macro. Cambodia Demographic & Health Survey 2000. Phnom Penh and Calverton, National Institute of Statistics, Directorate General for Health, and ORC Macro, 2001.
6. Sochantha T. *et al.* Insecticide-treated bed nets for the prevention of Plasmodium falciparum malaria in Cambodia: a cluster-randomised trial. *Tropical Medicine and International Health,* 2006, 11(8):1166-77.

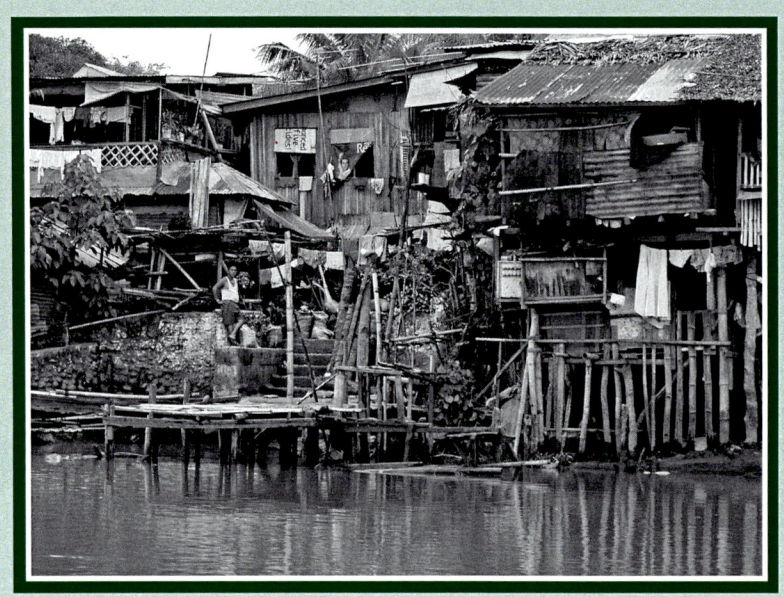

Public-private mix DOTS: a strategy to engage all health care providers in tuberculosis control and significantly increase access to DOTS services in the Philippines

Dr Michael N. Voniatis[1], Ms Lucille Nievera[1], Dr Jaime Y. Lagahid[2], Dr Rosalind G. Vianzon[2] Ms Amelia Sarmiento[3], Dr Charles Yu[4]

1. Summary

Public-Private Mix DOTS (PPMD) was adopted as a national strategy for the Philippines in 2003 to increase case detection and improve access to DOTS (directly observed treatment, short-course) services in poor urban areas by making greater use of private sector providers.[1] The Comprehensive and Unified Policy for Tuberculosis Control (CUP) was introduced the same year to enhance PPMD by unifying and harmonizing TB management by government agencies outside the public health sector. Between 2001 and 2004, the Philippine Coalition against Tuberculosis (PhilCAT) piloted five different PPMD models[4] and another 11 self-initiated PPMD units, all of which proved to be feasible and effective. The total number of PPMD units expected to be operating nationwide by the end of 2008 is 220, of which 170 are supported by the Global Fund to fight AIDS, Tuberculosis and Malaria (Global Fund). A 2005 World Health Organization (WHO) external evaluation showed that the units were effective and were providing quality DOTS services.[5]

The most recent results of PPMD strategy implementation are very encouraging, with an increase in case detection of 18% in implemented areas.[6] The treatment outcomes of PPMD units are at least equal to public sector performance.[6] About 5,000 private physicians throughout the country have been trained as DOTS referring physicians. The following mechanisms have been developed to improve the sustainability of PPMD:
- a monitoring and evaluation infrastructure;[8]
- a financial incentive—the TB-DOTS Out-patient Package, provided by the Philippine Health Insurance Corporation (PhilHealth);[9] and,
- local coalitions in support of PPMD.[10]

The PPMD strategy has so far proved effective and has been received well by the public. Its sustainability and further expansion to improve access by the urban poor and other marginalized populations to DOTS services will comprise measures of its overall success.

---

1 WHO Country Office in the Philippines, Manila, Philippines
2 National TB Program, National Center for Disease Prevention and Control, Dept. of Health, Manila, Philippines
3 Philippine Coalition Against Tuberculosis, Quezon Institute, Quezon City, Metro Manila, Philippines
4 Medical School, De La Salle University, Cavite, Philippines

2. Purpose

Using evidence from pilot projects, the PPMD strategy and the Comprehensive and Unified Policy for Tuberculosis Control (CUP) were developed as a way to expand DOTS beyond the public health sector and achieve tuberculosis (TB) control in a high burden country. The aim is to reduce tuberculosis prevalence and mortality by half by the year 2010. A significant proportion of people with TB symptoms were seeking care from the private sector,[16] but received inconsistent treatment and were not routinely reported.[29, 30] PPMD is an effective mode of TB control for the urban poor and other marginalized populations, and so addresses health equity issues. This paper explains how the PPMD strategy evolved and was implemented, as well as its effectiveness and scope for expansion.

2.1 Assumptions

The PPMD policy development process has been evidence-based. The policy is based on the following main assumptions:
1. The expansion of PPMD units by private organizations and NGOs can provide additional access to urban poor populations.
2. Advocacy, communication and social mobilization facilitate the removal of existing barriers to access to services at DOTS units.
3. Funding for TB control will be expanded through the greater use of the PhilHealth TB DOTS Outpatient package[14] by an increasing the number of PhilHealth-accredited DOTS units.

2.2 Process and history

Figure 1 shows the continuous process of development of the PPMD strategy. The initial concept of focusing on private physicians was based on earlier studies,[16,32] but the strategy was developed through piloting and modeling in the Philippines.

2.3 Background

Tuberculosis is a major killer disease in the Philippines, ranking sixth among leading causes of morbidity and mortality. It is estimated that 107 persons died of TB every day in 2005.[12] By the end of 2002, the public sector had introduced DOTS services in 100% of its health centres. However, the country was unable to reach the goal of achieving a 70% case detection rate for new smear positives.[17] A Joint Programme Review in 2002[18] concluded, among other things, that the country needed to make better use of the extensive private sector to accelerate progress towards the TB control targets.

The evidence for a public-private partnership in TB was fairly extensive.
- Tuberculosis is almost twice as prevalent among the urban poor as in the rest of the urban or rural population[13] and is two to three times more prevalent among those from the poorest than the richest income quintile of the population.[32]
- Among those with TB symptoms, 30% seek care from private physicians.[16]
- An estimated 30% of patients whose TB was unreported used the private sector.[16,31]

Figure 1: Development, establishment and expansion of PPMD in the Philippines

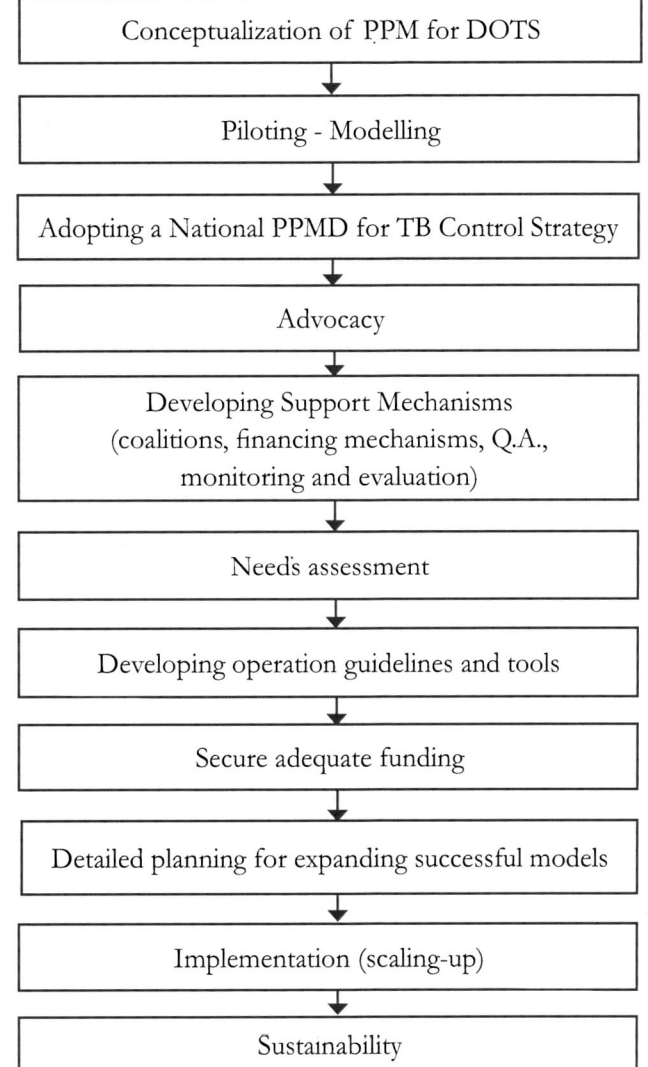

- An analysis of the TB drug market also provided evidence of the significant role of the private sector in TB management in the Philippines.[33]
- Treatment of TB by private physicians (1/3 of all cases) was inconsistent and variable, and some regimens prescribed did not conform to National TB Programme recommendations. [29,30]

PPMD was adopted as a national strategy in 2003, to increase case detection, harmonize TB management among health care providers, and increase overall access to DOTS services. In March 2003, the Comprehensive and Unified Policy for Tuberculosis Control was introduced to enhance PPMD and extend DOTS coverage. This did not replace the PPMD strategy, but gave it broader reach, potentially increasing its impact on health equity. The CUP aimed to coordinate TB patient management by government agencies beyond the public health sector, including academic institutions, NGOs, professional societies and the private sector.

Table 1: A brief history of TB control in the Philippines

1988:	First reference to public-private mix for TB control in the NTB Control Manual. [15]
1994:	Establishment of the Philippine Coalition Against Tuberculosis (PhilCAT).
1995:	Establishment of the first private DOTS clinic at the Santo Tomas University, Manila.
1996:	Introduction of DOTS strategy in the public sector.
1999:	Establishment of a private DOTS clinic at the Makati Medical Center, Metro Manila.
2001-2004:	Piloting by PhilCAT of the 5 CDC PPMD models.
2003:	Adoption and introduction by the Department of Health of the PPM for DOTS Strategy;
	Round 2 of the Global Fund to support PPMD.
	The Comprehensive and Unified Policy was signed by the President of the Philippines.
	DOTS certification and accreditation were introduced (Department of Health, PhilCAT, PhilHealth).
	PhiHealth TB DOTS outpatient benefit package was introduced.
2004:	Establishment of the National Coordinating Committee for PPMD.
	Operational Guidelines for PPMD developed, published and distributed.
	Scaling-up of PPMD through the Global Fund and the USAID PhilTIPS project.
	Two major evaluations showed PPMD was effective.
	Scaling-up of PPMD continues and expands to address the urban poor in Metro Manila.
	PPM DOTS made a component of the National Strategic Plan to Stop TB in the Philippines.
2007:	Another 50 PPMD units were installed (Round 5 of the Global Fund), reaching a total of 170 PPMD units.
2008:	Remaining 50 PPMD units under the Global Fund Round 5 implemented.

Box 1: Types of PPMD units

There are two types of PPMD units in the Philippines. The first type is a public DOTS facility that already accepts walk-in patients, but has made agreements with private physicians who have been trained in DOTS and will refer their TB patients for diagnosis and treatment (case holding and directly-observed treatment, or DOT).

The other type is a privately-owned and -run facility that will become a DOTS centre. The health staff that run the facility are trained to function as DOTS providers and do sputum smear microscopy. Once the units are established, they also accept referrals from private physicians as well as walk-in patients for diagnosis and treatment (case holding and DOT). These privately-owned PPMD units can be regarded as additional DOTS centres, thereby improving access, whereas the public PPMD units can improve TB reporting and case management.

2.4 Political climate, stakeholders, and policy-making

Despite economic development, a significant proportion of the population in the Philippines still lives below the poverty line, particularly in urban areas.[12] The urban poor comprise up to 45% of the total population in parts of Metro Manila. The Government recognizes that the failure to effectively reduce the spread and prevalence of a major disease like TB can roll back many of the recent economic gains.

Political support for PPMD is shown by the fact the Department of Health has never decreased the annual budget for TB control, and has increased it somewhat in recent years.[20] The budget for TB at the central level (in the Department of Health) has doubled for 2008. At the local implementation level, the political response has been variable but, in most instances, positive to the PPMD strategy. The financing of the PPMD strategy is secured through 2011, to a large extent through Rounds 2 and 5 of the Global Fund, but the overall long-term sustainability of PPMD units will depend on other factors, including health insurance reimbursements.

Advocacy has played a big role in the acceptance and implementation of the PPMD strategy. The Philippine Coalition against Tuberculosis has been the major ally of Department of Health in this endeavour. It has mobilized leaders from the public and private sectors and advocated to local chief executives, professional societies, and communities. This initial advocacy, which started well before the official adoption of the PPMD strategy, has been a major part of the process for establishing a PPMD unit (see Figure 2).[1]

Figure 2: Model Process
(The Fishbone Process)

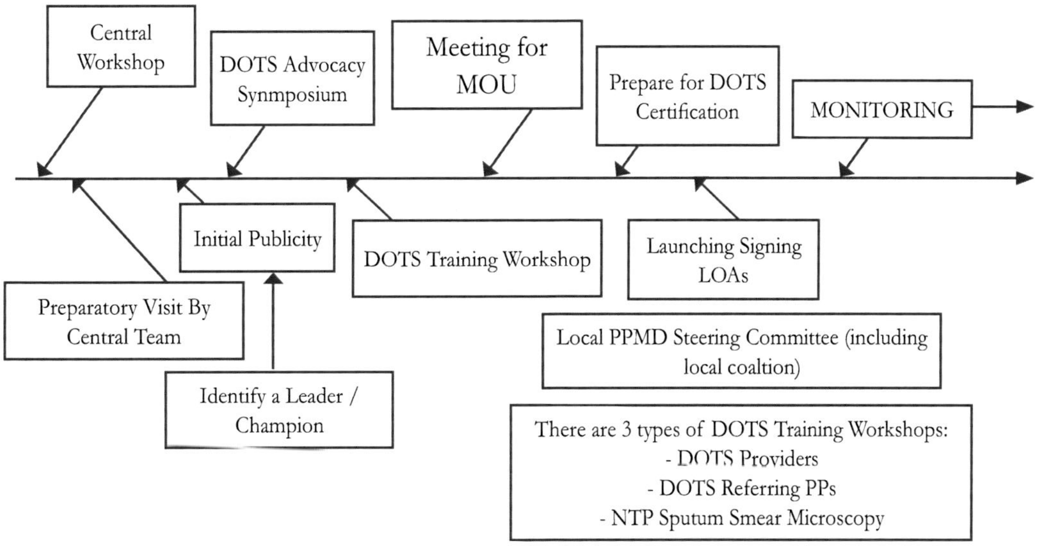

An initial symposium was held for stakeholders from the public health sector, private physicians, professional societies, local chief executives, local NGOs and academic institutions. Leaders and allies were identified, and these formed a core group to advocate to private physicians to be trained for PPMD, and also campaign for the engagement of local government units in increasing enrolment of the poor in PhilHealth.[5]

Advocacy with private sector physicians for PPMD was effective for the following reasons:
- The DOTS strategy for the management of TB in the public sector had already proved successful, gaining a reputation for quality services with excellent outcomes through the provision of good quality TB drugs.[11]

---

5 PhilHealth is a government health insurance scheme that aims to provide substantial financing for health care at primary, secondary and tertiary levels. Most members are government employees, private company employees, or poor persons enrolled by the local government.

- TB drugs were to be provided free to all patients treated under DOTS in both the public and private sectors. TB drugs in the private sector are expensive and not affordable for most patients.
- PPMD leaders and champions had emerged in both the private and public sectors.[25]
- It was expected that the PhilHealth TB DOTS Outpatient Package would reimburse adequate funds to both private DOTS-referring physicians and private DOTS providers, including a referral fee and subsequent consultation fees during the clinical follow up of DOTS patients.[1]

2.5 Enabling factors

The Department of Health shared the burden of PPMD implementation with PhilCAT, an experienced partner in PPMD advocacy and implementation. No significant changes were necessary in the Department of Health administration to implement the strategy, and substantial funding came from the Global Fund and the United States Agency for International Development (USAID). The National TB Programme hired four additional staff and set up an integrated structure for the monitoring and supervision of PPMD, with a National Coordinating Committee and 16 Regional Coordinating Committees. The regional committees employed one Nurse-Coordinator and one secretary each, but the national committee had no additional staff. Additional staff at all levels are funded through the Global Fund. The total external amount invested in the PPMD strategy in the Philippines over the last five years is approximately US$ 16 million. The PhilHealth TB DOTS Outpatient package was specifically developed for the financial support and sustainability of the PPMD strategy.

2.6 Additional effects of PPMD policy

Communication of information to the population about the fight against TB and the availability of free treatment resulted in synergies, evident from the increase in case detection that occurred in both PPMD and corresponding public health centres.[5] The availability of external funding made it possible to effectively introduce and scale up the strategy. It also helped in improving the overall monitoring and supervision of both PPMD units and those in the public sector.

In addition, the introduction and expansion of PPMD led to improved DOTS implementation overall. The regular national DOTS programme was strengthened through joint training, advocacy, communication and social mobilization, and through joint monitoring and supervisory activities at all levels. PPMD did not crowd out funding for or result in the downgrading or elimination of other Department of Health programmes, including those for maternal and child health, malaria control, sexually transmitted infections and HIV/AIDS.

PPMD opened the door increased involvement by local government units in TB control, since local government units are the health care payers, following health system devolution in the Philippines. PPMD also helped build local coalitions and partnerships.[4] A number of NGOs and corporations became interested in the approach and some have implemented the PPMD strategy in the workplace.[21]

2.7 Difficulties in implementation

For the local government units, the challenge of implementing PPMD lay in: ensuring access to comprehensive DOTS services; mobilizing adequate financing for TB services for the poor; strengthening the existing public health infrastructure; and strengthening existing human resources. Their support to PPMD was uneven, with shortfalls in staff, particularly medical technologists. Other local government agencies beyond the health sector also encountered difficulties in implementing the Comprehensive and Unified Policy. These stemmed from the lack of awareness of some local chief executives about the social value of the DOTS and PPMD strategies, and similarly of the concerned communities and the NGOs working with them. Some local government units failed to support enrolment of the poor in PhilHealth or to remit TB Outpatient Package reimbursements to the public PPMD units for TB patients enrolled under the scheme. Some private physicians, who might have been keys to reaching the urban poor, were hesitant to participate. Several small local NGOs had limited capacity to deliver quality services using the strategy and regarded the initiative as an opportunity to obtain funding.

Low enrolment in PhilHealth by the poor limits revenues for PPMD operations and endangers their financial sustainability, particularly for the wholly privately-owned ones. Although all PPMD units receive free TB drugs from the Department of Health, they still have to cover their operational costs for sputum microscopy services and directly observed treatment.

2.8 Using evidence to improve implementation of PPMD

Since its official introduction in 2003, the PPMD strategy has been expanded rapidly, particularly following the approval of Rounds 2 and 5 of the Global Fund and the USAID-supported Philippine Tuberculosis Initiative for the Private Sector (PhilTIPS).

Evidence for the success or otherwise of the PPMD strategy was obtained through the following special studies, evaluations and assessments, as well as routine data collection and information:
- 2004: Evaluation of effectiveness of the 5 PPMD Centers for Disease Control (CDC) model units[4]
- 2004-2005: Economic analysis of non-Global Fund PPMD units in Metro Manila[19]
- Early 2005: WHO external evaluation of the first 7 PPMD units established with Global Fund support
- 2006: Final evaluation of PhilTIPS[21]
- 2006: PhilCAT used a routine monitoring and evaluation system for all Global Fund-supported PPMD units; by 2007, it included all PPMD units operating in the country under all initiatives.
- 2006: Needs assessment for improving access to DOTS in Metro Manila[12]

Following the Department of Health's official adoption and introduction of the PPMD strategy in 2003, the final evaluation of the five PPMD pilot models in diverse private facilities in 2004 showed satisfactory results.[4] The economic analysis in Metro Manila[19] showed that

PPMD units had been effective in significantly increasing case detection, had reached an average treatment success rate of 85% (equal to the global target of 85% and very close to the public sector performance of 88%), and were used primarily by very poor patients. The final evaluation of PhilTIPS in 2006[7] showed that their PPMD units provided 100% supervised treatment and had a treatment success rate of 87%. There was very high patient satisfaction with regard to comfort, availability of educational materials, and accessibility of clinics.

The WHO Philippines country office, the Japan International Cooperation Agency (JICA)-supported TB Project and the Department of Health carried out an assessment of the TB control performance of each of the 17 municipalities of Metro Manila in early 2006.[12] The assessment showed variable performance, finding coverage by the public sector insufficient in most of the municipalities, in terms of the number of DOTS units per population. It also found that most public DOTS centres offered only clinic-based DOT services.

The assessment analyzed municipality-wise weaknesses as well. For example, Quezon City, with a population of 2.5 million, had too few microscopy centres to adequately diagnose and follow up cases, resulting in a low case notification rate and poor treatment outcomes. Based on these criteria, the assessment found that at least half the population of Metro Manila had inadequate access to DOTS services at public sector or PPMD units. The report suggested specific remedial measures for each municipality. In response, more private and NGO PPMD units were established, particularly in Quezon City. Advocacy with local chief executives was been carried on with some success, and, direct sputum smear microscopy was strengthened in Quezon City through the JICA-supported quality improvement project for TB, with improvements seen in treatment outcomes.

Monitoring, supervision and evaluation of the technical aspects of the PPMD strategy are done using the Electronic TB Register, a standardized monitoring tool implemented by PhilCAT. This tool is validated by regularly comparing the monitored data to TB registers from the PPMD units.

The equity aspects of the PPMD strategy have not yet been adequately researched, but socio-economic and employment status have been assessed in special studies,[4,19] and additional indicators of equity and access were developed[12,35] and will be integrated into routine monitoring.

3. Main achievements of PPMD strategy

The main achievements of the PPMD strategy are summarized below.

a. Increase in detection of new smear-positive cases: In the 70 PPMD units established under support from Round 2 of the Global Fund, the number of new smear-positive TB cases detected by PPMD (cumulative) increased by an average of 18%[6] from April to June 2007. An increase in case detection was also observed as early as 2005, during the WHO external evaluation of PPMD units funded by the Global Fund.[5] The increase in the detection of new smear positive cases reached 8% after one year of implementation of the strategy, with an additional 10.4% increase in case detection by the public sector.

b. Achieving satisfactory treatment success rates: Monitoring data[6] from the 70 PPMD units operating with support from Round 2 of the Global Fund showed a treatment success rate of 88%, which is close to performance under the National TB Programme, even though most PPMD patients are under directly- observed treatment with a family member as the designated treatment partner, rather than the non-family member usually recommended. [36] Similar outcomes related to 2-month sputum conversion rates were found in the WHO external evaluation, with all PPMD units exceeding 85%. In other words, the PPMD strategy succeeded in meeting its objective to provide quality DOTS services.

c. Engagement of health care providers: One indicator for assessing the successful implementation of PPMD is the actual participation of the private sector. A WHO external evaluation[5] found the proportion of actively engaged private sector providers, compared to those who were DOTS-referring, to be 57.5% (average of seven pilot areas in Metro Manila.) More recent monitoring data[6] from the 70 PPMD units operating with Global Fund support show that the actual number of participating private physicians (1,119) exceeded the target of 840. This included only active participation, defined as referral of a minimum of one patient with TB symptoms to a PPMD unit per quarter. The engagement of referring private physicians has progressed beyond simply obtaining DOTS training, and even includes formal contractual relationships with PPMD units.[6]

d. Accessibility of PPMD to low-income patients and patient satisfaction: Information on access by various income and social groups to PPMD has not been collected routinely, but only through special studies. Income analysis of over 300 patients showed that their mean monthly household income was US$ 214[19] (or US$ 1.40 per day per capita), compared to the average monthly household income of US$ 1696 in Metro Manila, using current prices.

Closely related to improved access is patients' satisfaction or perceived quality of the services provided.[22] The same study quoted in the preceding paragraph looked at why patients used PPMD units. Their responses, ranked by frequency, included the availability of: free drugs (77.4%), free consultation (60.4%) and free examination (52.5%). A 2006 evaluation[7] of PhilTIPS, which ran 20 private sector PPMD units, reported very high satisfaction in all respects (a 97% average rating), with equally high rates of complete and supervised treatment, and an average treatment success rate of 87%. In general, privately-operated PPMD units outperform public PPMD units, both in case detection and in treatment outcomes. Private PPMD units serve more TB patients[6] than public sector units. This indicates that the quality assurance component of PPMD is working well in the private sector.[6]

e. **Communication with stakeholders:** The pilot PPMD sites and PHilCAT maintain a strong partnership with the National TB Programme and the Department of Health at the central level. Perhaps as a result, the PPMD strategy is now regarded as a strategy that can successfully reduce barriers to access to services faced by the urban poor and other marginalized populations, such as travel costs to clinics and opening times of public DOTS clinics.[12] The relationships between the pilot sites and the local government units and other stakeholders are in the early stages of their development.

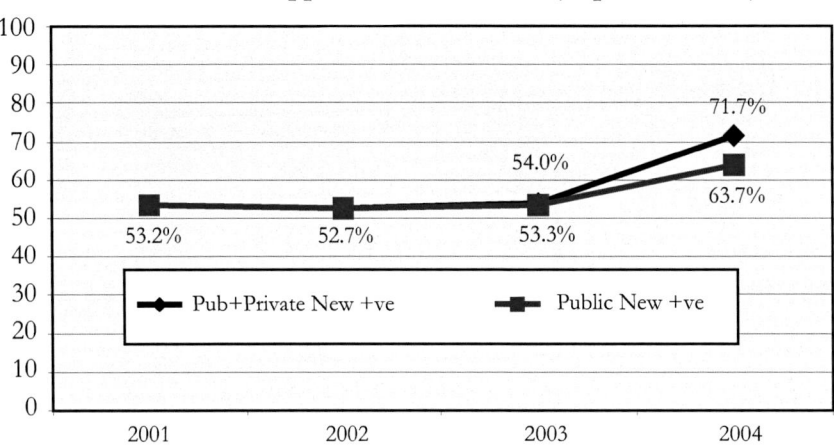

Figure 3: Case Detection Rate
All GFATM supported PPMD Units (Pop. 2.9 million)

Planning, implementation, progress made and lessons learned from the PPMD experience have been regularly shared with stakeholders from public and private sectors in programme implementation reviews, planning workshops, and the National TB Programme Consultative Workshops. Lessons learned were also presented at the annual PhilCAT Convention and posters on PPMD implementation were presented at the international and regional meetings of the International Union against Tuberculosis and Lung Disease.

4. Conclusions

The evidence gathered on the PPMD experience so far is limited to process, output and outcome indicators. Its impact on the disease can be assessed only once the urban poor are fully covered by the PPMD strategy and the CUP has been effectively implemented, engaging at least 90% of all health care providers.

The PPMD strategy's ambitious initial objectives related to increased case detection and treatment success rate have been achieved,[6] and the response from health care providers has been very positive.[6,23] The strategy has been found to be effective in improving access by the urban poor to DOTS services[12] and to free TB drugs.[19] This finding is consistent with the experience with PPMD strategies in other countries, such as India.[35] Adequate funding from the Global Fund and the significant experience of PhilCAT in implementing the strategy helped make it a success.

The Comprehensive and Unified Policy for Tuberculosis Control has been less successful, because of incomplete commitment of stakeholders outside the public health structure and the lack of availability of sufficient funds beyond the regular government budget for its implementation.[20]

4.1 Challenges and lessons learned

Despite the successful implementation of the PPMD strategy and the partial implementation of the CUP, significant challenges remain. Key among these are the following:

- Both PPMD and the CUP need to be expanded to meet equity goals. Implementation of the PPMD strategy has been able to achieve the technical and epidemiological TB control targets. Implementation of the CUP has been more fragmented and it does not cover all prisons, all government agencies and all public hospitals. A better approach to measuring outcomes and impact is needed to demonstrate the contribution of the PPMD and CUP to improvements in health equity.
- PPMD needs to be institutionalized, to ensure its political, financial and socio-cultural sustainability. Implementation of the strategy has so far relied on external funding, mainly from the Global Fund.
- Implementation of the PhilHealth TB DOTS Outpatient Package throughout the country is critical, since this contributes 50% to 100% of the financial requirements in a significant proportion of PPMD units.[28] PhilHealth certification and accreditation will be needed for all DOTS units, to achieve universal coverage.
- The momentum achieved in 2003 in advocating for the PPMD strategy needs to be maintained and used to address equity through increased geographical coverage. This will require the strengthening and nationwide expansion of TB coalitions.
- Expansion of both PPMD and the CUP requires the participation of all health care providers. This means that about 10,000 private physicians, and some of those working in government hospitals, will need to be trained in DOTS nationwide.
- Finally, securing adequate funding to expand the PPMD strategy to all urban poor and marginalized populations remains a challenge.

These challenges can be overcome using the experience gained. Specifically:
- Commitment and leadership from both the private and public sector are essential for the successful initiation and implementation of PPMD.[25] Appropriate selection criteria (leadership and commitment, adequate population, and an adequate mass of private practitioners) lead to a successful PPMD unit.[6]
- Local TB coalitions, representing both the public and private sectors at the local level play a significant role in advocacy with local chief executives, private physicians, professional societies and communities.[26]
- Assuring the quality of PPMD contributes to its success and sustainability and facilitates advocacy, private sector participation and support from local chief executives.[1]
- Good publicity when launching PPMD can increase the use of public DOTS facilities.[5]
- Use of evidence, especially if locally derived, is important in convincing key opinion leaders to change behaviors among physicians.
- Support from local governments contributes to success and sustainability.[28]

4.2 The future of PPMD

Existing PPMD workplans extend to the end of 2008. It is hoped that the PPMD strategy will be expanded over the next five years to fully cover the urban poor and other marginalized populations and to engage all health care providers in the country.

The PPMD strategy is currently implemented in a top-down manner, but simplifying the process will require the training of private DOTS-referring physicians and the establishment of PPMD units from existing public DOTS-certified and -accredited units. Such a bottom-up approach will rely on advocacy with local government units, and strong partnership with local TB coalitions.

It is reasonable to expect that the public-private mix concept will be used in other domains of TB control, like the management of multi-drug resistant TB, TB/HIV coinfection and TB in children. Other public health programmes, such as those to control malaria and HIV/AIDS, are currently studying the possibility of introducing a public-private mix strategy. The original spirit of PPMD has been maintained in its scaling up, with new partners becoming interested in joining forces to expand the strategy for the benefit of the urban poor in Metro Manila.[28]

Endnotes

1. Philippine Coalition against Tuberculosis and Department of Health. *Operational guidelines for public-private mix DOTS in the Philippines*. Manila, PhilCAT, 2004.
2. Republic of the Philippines. *Executive order no.187: Instituting a comprehensive and unified policy for TB control in the Philippines*. Manila, Government of the Philippines, 2003.
3. World Health Organization. *Involving private practitioners in tuberculosis control: issues, interventions and emerging policy framework*. WHO, Geneva, 2001.
4. Centers for Disease Prevention and Control. Joint PPMD pilot project evaluation. Manila, Atlanta, CDC, 2004.
5. World Health Organization Regional Office for the Western Pacific. *External evaluation of public-private mix DOTS under the Global Fund-supported project in the Philippines*. Manila, WHO, 2005.
6. Philippine Coalition against Tuberculosis. Quarterly monitoring reports Q14 and Q15, under the Global Fund-supported PPMD project. Manila, PhilCAT, 2007.
7. Philippine Tuberculosis Initiatives for Private Sector. Final report on the implementation of PPMD in the private sector. Manila, PhilTIPS, USAID, 2006.
8. Philippine Coalition against Tuberculosis and Department of Health. *Operational guidelines for public-private mix DOTS in the Philippines*. Manila, PhilCAT, 2004.
9. Philippine Health Insurance Corporation. *The TB DOTS out-patient benefit package*. Manila, PhilHealth, 2003.
10. Philippine Coalition against Tuberculosis. *Guidebook on local TB coalition building and strengthening*. Manila, PhilCAT, 2006.
11. WHO. WHO Report 2006: Global tuberculosis control: surveillance, planning, financing. Geneva, WHO, 2006.
12. WHO Philippines. Mapping the urban poor in Metro Manila and improving their access to DOTS services (draft). Manila, WHO Country Office in the Philippines, 2006.
13. Tupasi T.E. *et al*. Tuberculosis in the urban poor settlements in the Philippines. *Int J Tuberc Lung Dis*, 2000, 4(1):4-11.
14. Philippine Health Insurance Corporation. *The TB DOTS out-patient benefit package*. Manila, PhilHealth, 2003.
15. Department of Health. *Manual for the national tuberculosis control program*. Manila, Government of the Philippines, 1988:12.
16. Tupasi T.E. *et al*. The 1997 nationwide tuberculosis prevalence survey in the Philippines. *Int J Tuberc Lung Dis*, 1999, 3(6):471-477.
17. WHO. WHO Report 2004: Global tuberculosis control: surveillance, planning, financing", Geneva, WHO, 2004.
18. World Health Organization, Regional Office for the Western Pacific. *Joint programme review of the Philippine TB control programme*. ,Manila, WHO, 2002.
19. Voniatis M.N. *et al*. Economic analysis of public-private mix DOTS in Metro Manila. Poster presentation at 26th International Conference on Lung Health, IUATLD, Paris, 2005.

20. Department of Health. *National strategic plan to stop TB 2006-2010, Philippines*. Manila, Government of the Philippines, 2006.
21. Philippine Tuberculosis Initiatives for Private Sector. *Managing tuberculosis in the workplace: a guide for companies implementing DOTS*. Manila, PhilTIPS, Philippine Business for Social Progress, USAID and Department of Health, 2005.
22. Tuberculosis Coalition for Technical Assistance. *International standards for tuberculosis care (ISTC)*. The Hague, Tuberculosis Coalition for Technical Assistance, 2006.
23. Philippine Tuberculosis Initiatives for Private Sector. *Best practices and approaches in public-private mix DOTS*. Manila, PhilTIPS, USAID, 2006.
24. United States Agency for International Development. *Guide for DOTS certification assessors*. Manila, Philippine Tuberculosis Initiatives for Private Sector, USAID, 2004.
25. Voniatis M.N. Mission report on public-private mix DOTS monitoring and supervision. Manila, WHO Western Pacific Regional Office, 2003.
26. Philippine Coalition against Tuberculosis. *Guidebook on local TB coalition building and strengthening*. Manila, PhilCAT, 2006.
27. Sarriot E.G. *et al*. Qualitative research to make practical sense of sustainability in primary health care projects implemented by non-governmental organizations. *Int J Health Plann Mgmt*, 2004, 19:3–22.
28. Philippine Coalition against Tuberculosis. PPMD programme implementation reviews. 4-20 September 2007 (draft). Manila, PhilCAT, 2007.
29. Portero L.J. and M.Rubio. Private practitioners and tuberculosis control in the Philippines: strangers when they meet? *Tropical Medicine and International Health*, 2003, 8:329-35.
30. Auer C. *et al*. Diagnosis and management of tuberculosis by private practitioners in Manila, Philippines. *Health Policy*, 2006, 77:172-81.
31. Philippine Coalition against Tuberculosis. *Current trends in TB management by private physicians in the Philippines: a survey in five private health settings*. Manila, PhilCAT, 2002.
32. Peabody J.W. *et al*. The burden of disease, economic costs and clinical consequences of tuberculosis in the Philippines. *Health Policy and Planning*, 2005, 20(6):347-53.
33. World Health Organization. Analysis of drug market in 5 high TB burden countries. Geneva, WHO, 2002.
34. World Health Organization Green Light Committee. Report of the 6th monitoring visit at the DOTS-plus project at Makati Medical Center/Tropical Disease Foundation, Philippines. Geneva, WHO Green Light Committee, 2005.
35. World Health Organization. *Cost and cost-effectiveness of public-private mix: evidence from two pilot projects in India*. Geneva, WHO, 2004.
36. Department of Health. *Manual of procedures for TB control in the Philippines*. Manila, Government of the Philippines, 2005.
37. *Manila Standard*, 7/11/2006.

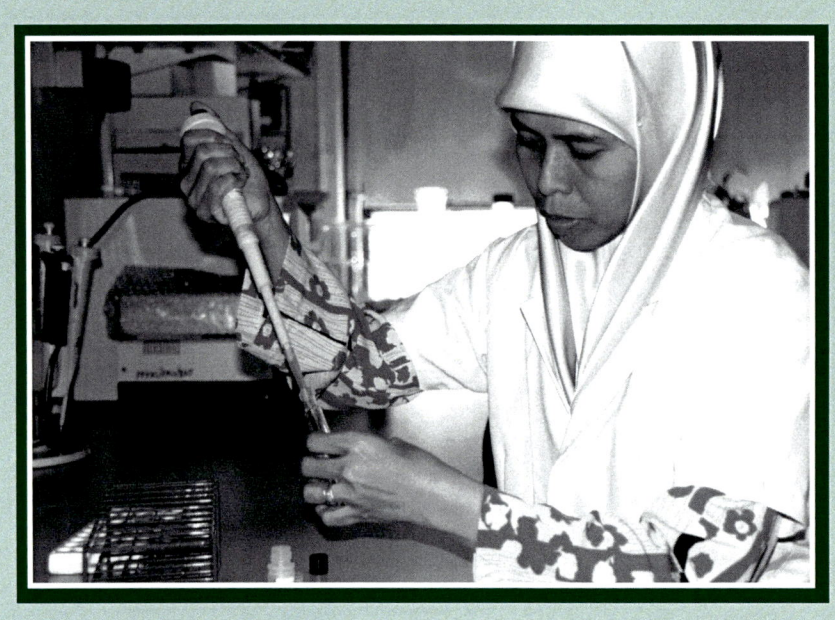

Geographic equity in distribution of scarce dialysis resources in Malaysia

Lim Teck Onn[1], Adrian Goh[1]

1. Summary

Dialysis is renal replacement therapy that replaces normal kidney function by artificial means and is an indicated treatment for end stage renal failure. It is an effective but costly life support treatment that, without government funding, is unaffordable for most Malaysians. This case study asks how the Ministry of Health should address the issue of equity in access to dialysis.

Historically, dialysis was a highly inaccessible treatment in Malaysia. Dialysis provision accelerated in the 1990s, following high demand for dialysis treatment and increasing public financing as the economy grew rapidly from the late 1980s onwards. Growth in access to the treatment has been greater in the economically advanced states, however, while the poorer states continue to lag behind in treatment provision.

Concentration indices (represented by the symbol C) show that, although the geographic distribution of dialysis is unequally distributed towards the well-off states, the extent of inequality has declined from 0.11 in 1997 to 0.05 in 2004. From 1997 to 2004, government dialysis has gone from favouring the well-off states (C=0.037) to favouring the poorer states (C= -0.047). At the same time, although the charitable and private sectors continue to be distributed towards the economically advantaged states, they have reduced the extent of inequality towards the poorer states. The distribution of dialysis confirms our expectation that the private sector has concentrated its facilities in economically developed states, while the public sector places more emphasis on the poorer states in accordance with its social equity mission.

Malaysia's experience as a middle income developing country in providing expensive dialysis shows that it is possible to ensure the equality of access to a scarce therapy, even in a situation where the benefits of economic growth are not equally distributed. The relative decline in public sector services does not inevitably have a negative impact on equity, if public sector services are targeted to areas where private sector provision is unprofitable.

2. Problem definition

How should the Ministry of Health, as the regulator and major funder of health care in Malaysia, address the issue of equity in access to dialysis services?

---

1   Clinical Research Centre, Ministry of Health Malaysia

Where equity refers to horizontal equity of access to care or "equal access for equal need,"[1] equity is defined by the World Health Organization as follows[2]:

"Equity is the absence of avoidable or remediable differences among groups of people, whether those groups are defined…geographically."

2.1 Introduction and brief history

Dialysis is a form of therapy that replaces normal kidney function by artificial means and is indicated for patients suffering from end stage renal disease. Left untreated, end stage renal disease is uniformly fatal within a year of onset. Dialysis is an effective life support treatment and depending on age and health status of the patient, it can prolong life on treatment for up to 30 years in Malaysia.

In general, there are two modalities of dialysis treatment:

1. Haemodialysis is a machine-based treatment where dialysis is carried out across an artificial membrane housed in a dialyser connected to the patient's arterio-venous fistula via an extra corporeal circuit. In Malaysia, almost all patients undergo three sessions of haemodialysis per week with each session lasting for four to five hours. Haemodialysis can be delivered as a centre-based therapy, where the patient attends a dialysis facility for treatment or as a home-based therapy, where the haemodialysis machine is installed at home (or even at a place of work) where the patient performs the treatment.
2. Continuous ambulatory peritoneal dialysis is a process where dialysis is performed across the natural peritoneal membrane in the abdomen via a permanent catheter. After several hours during which dialysis occurs, the dialysate is drained out via the same catheter and fresh dialysate infused for another cycle (one exchange) of dialysis. Patients typically undergo four exchanges per day. Continuous ambulatory peritoneal dialysis is a home-based therapy and the patient is required to follow-up with a nephrologist on a regular basis.

Kidney transplantation is the alternative and preferred treatment for end stage renal disease. However, due to the shortage of organ donors in Malaysia, dialysis will remain the main form of treatment in the foreseeable future, with haemodialysis as the most common dialysis modality.

Unfortunately, dialysis is an expensive treatment. In 2004, it cost the Government RM 33,642 (US$ 8,800) to provide a patient with one year of haemodialysis and RM 31,635 (US$ 8,300) for continuous ambulatory peritoneal dialysis at a Ministry of Health centre, about double the gross domestic product (GDP) per capita of RM 17,644 (US$ 4,600). Without subsidization, dialysis, treatment would not be affordable for most of the population.

2.2 Dialysis in Malaysia

As of 2005, Malaysia has 13,337 patients on dialysis at a rate of 510 per million population (pmp) while 3,054 new cases were accepted into dialysis (at a rate of 117 pmp).

As Figure 1 and Table 1 show, dialysis remained a highly inaccessible treatment until the 1990s, except for the fortunate few. Indeed, there were no dialysis centres at all outside of Kuala Lumpur until 1984 and, even then, only in large towns and cities. Such was the mismatch between the need for and availability of dialysis that the Ministry of Health's guideline for prioritizing access to dialysis services in the early 1980s was based on the following criteria, in descending order of priority: (a) patients with acute renal failure; (b) patients being prepared for transplant from a living related donor; (c) patients with failed graft following living related donor transplant; (d) government employees and their dependants.

Figure 1: Renal replacement therapy and income, 1980-2005

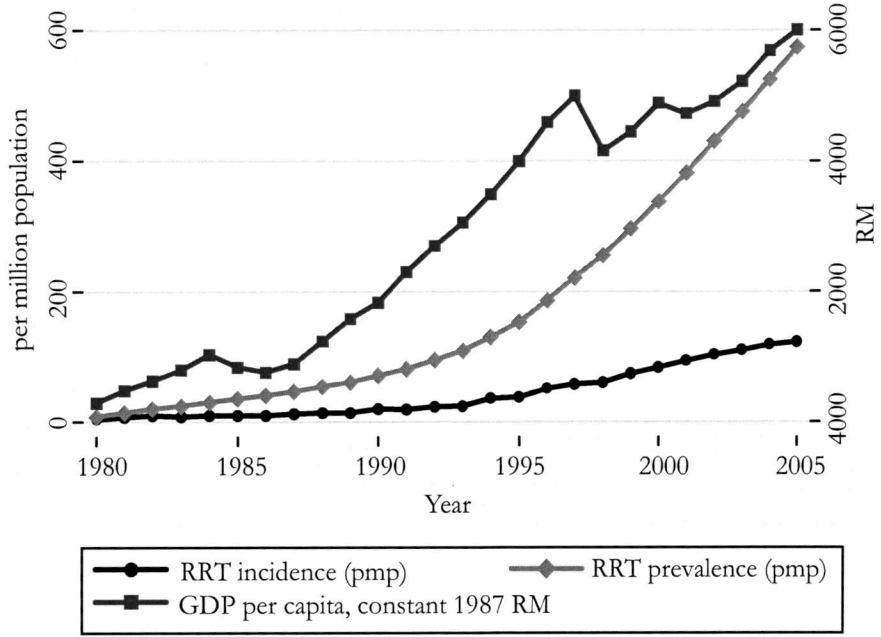

Sources: Malaysian National Renal Registry. Annual reports of the Malaysian Dialysis and Transplant Registry 2003-2007[4], IMF World Economic Outlook Database.[5]

Table 1: Trend of dialysis provision in Malaysia (pmp), 1980-2005

	1980	1985	1990	1995	2000	2004	2005
Renal replacement therapy incidence	4	10	20	38	84	119	123
Renal replacement therapy prevalence	8	35	71	153	338	525	574
Dialysis incidence	2	7	13	33	78	112	117
Dialysis prevalence	4	26	46	108	285	463	510

Source: Malaysian National Renal Registry. Annual reports of the Malaysian Dialysis and Transplant Registry 2003-2007.[4]

The growth in dialysis provision began to accelerate in the 1990s, as Malaysia entered a period of sustained high economic growth from the late 1980s onwards. Although public demand for dialysis treatment grew in tandem with increasing affluence, the public and private sectors were unable to meet the increased demand for the service. In response, the dialysis sector was liberalized by allowing non-governmental organizations (NGOs) to operate dialysis centres and approving the establishment of dialysis facilities without requiring an on-site nephrologist or, in some cases, a medical doctor.

Today, three types of providers offer dialysis services in Malaysia: the government (public) sector, the private sector and the charitable (NGO) sector. Public sector services comprise dialysis units in Ministry of Health hospitals, at university hospitals of the Ministry of Education, and at military hospitals and health facilities operated by the Ministry of Defence.

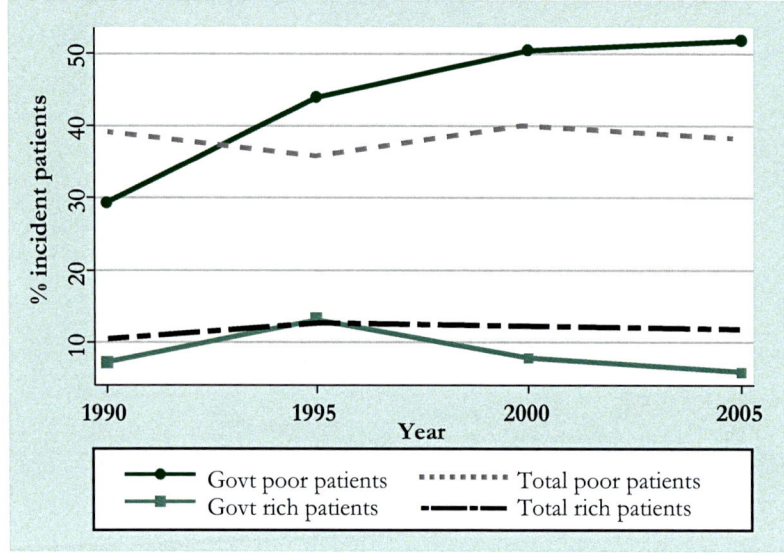

Figure 2: Incident patients by income group, 1990-2005

Source: Malaysian National Renal Registry. Annual reports of the Malaysian Dialysis and Transplant Registry 2003-2007.[4]

The Ministry of Health centres tend to provide dialysis services for active and retired civil servants and their dependents, the poor, and those living in areas where other dialysis providers are not available. As Figure 2 shows, the government dialysis sector enrols a larger proportion of poor patients (those earning less than RM 1000 per month).

Private sector dialysis includes stand-alone centres and facilities attached to private hospitals, and tends to serve employer-funded patients, privately-insured patients and those affluent enough to be self-funded.

The charitable (NGO) sector is a type of dialysis provider probably unique to Malaysia and Singapore. These centres are operated by the National Kidney Foundation, social service organizations like the Rotary and Lions clubs, and religious bodies. Patients are funded through public donations and some government subsidies. These services act as a safety net for those who are unable to be accepted into the public programme[2] or are unable to afford private dialysis.

---

2   This may be the case, for example, when government centres cannot accept more patients.

Much of the recent growth in dialysis services has been driven by growth in the private and charitable sectors, indicated by the declining share of patients served by government centres, as Figure 3 shows.

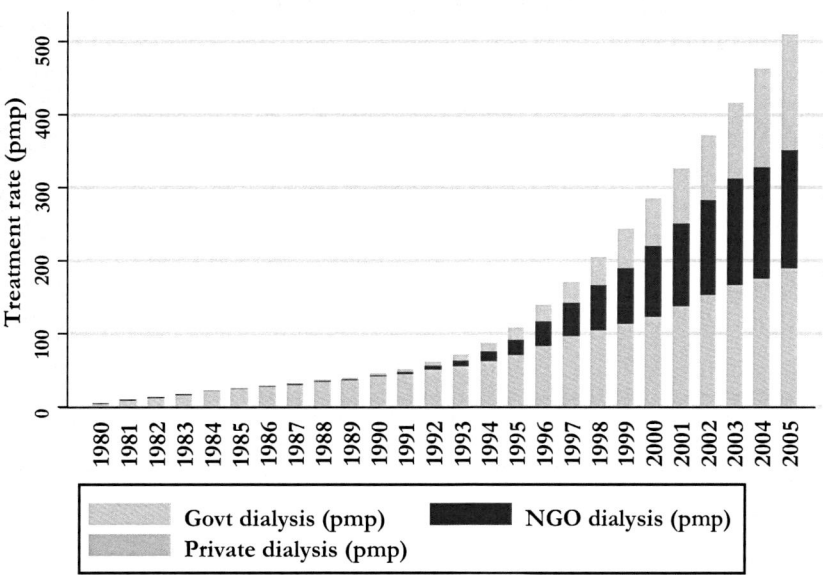

Figure 3: Dialysis treatment by sector (pmp) 1980-2005

Source: Malaysian National Renal Registry. Annual reports of the Malaysian Dialysis and Transplant Registry 2003-2007[4].

Government funding of dialysis directly or indirectly accounted for 67% of patients on dialysis in 2005. As Table 2 shows, the share of patients funded by the Government has declined in the 1990s, along with the decline in the public sector's share of dialysis provision. However, from the late 1990s, a series of public finance policies led to increasing public support for dialysis and eventually returned the public share to about two-third of total funding. In the 1990s, funding by charity has increased in tandem with its enhanced role as a treatment provider. While a significant proportion of patients are self-funded, both these sources (funding by charity and self-funding) declined relatively from the late 1990s, as greater public financing became available.

Table 2: Funding for dialysis(% patients), 1980-2005

Financing for dialysis by sector, 2005 RM million (%)	1990		1995		2000		2005	
• Public	15.4	(64)	39.4	(56)	92.2	(46)	255.2	(67)
• Charity	0.6	(3)	5.3	(8)	29.2	(14)	45.3	(12)
• Private	7.9	(33)	25.5	(36)	81.0	(41)	78.6	(21)
Total funding	23.9	(100)	70.2	(100)	202.4	(100)	379.1	(100)

Source: Malaysian National Renal Registry. Annual reports of the Malaysian Dialysis and Transplant Registry 2003-2007[4].

2.3 Brief history of dialysis in Malaysia

The private sector pioneered chronic dialysis treatment for end-stage renal function in Malaysia in 1966, when public donations enabled the purchase of an "artificial kidney" machine to treat end-stage renal function, following wide press coverage of the plight of a patient in Kuala Lumpur. From here, haemodialysis provision spread to the Ministry of Health Kuala Lumpur Hospital in 1969 and to other states, starting in 1984. By the late 1980s, the Ministry of Health began implementing a programme to establish haemodialysis units in all state general hospitals and later in large district hospitals. By the end of 2005, over 400 dialysis centres of both modalities were functioning in the country, including 137 haemodialysis centres in Ministry of Health hospitals, including those in small, remote districts.

Table 3: Timeline of expansion in dialysis provision in Malaysia

Date	Event	Remarks
1966	1st chronic haemodialysis facility established in a private charitable hospital near Kuala Lumpur	Machine funded through public donations following press coverage of the plight of a patient
1969	1st public sector haemodialysis facility with 18 patients established at the Kuala Lumpur Hospital	
1970	National Kidney Foundation launched	Training & public education
Early 1970s	Corporate dialysis centres for their staff	Services provided in Kuala Lumpur only
1979	Home haemodialysis programme where patients who could afford to purchase their own haemodialysis machines and consumables could dialyse at home after training at Kuala Lumpur Hospital.	Up to 350 patients on home haemodialysis at its peak, but now largely superseded by centre haemodialysis
1984	Six haemodialysis units established outside Kuala Lumpur	Partly funded by a donation from the Association of Cabinet Ministers' Wives
1984	Continuous ambulatory peritoneal dialysis introduced in Kuala Lumpur Hospital	
1993	First National Kidney Foundation dialysis centre in Kuala Lumpur	In collaboration with the Social Welfare Ministry and partly funded by a Broadcasting Ministry telethon
1996	Finance Ministry pledge a RM 25 million grant to National Kidney Foundation	
2001	Government subsidy for deserving patients dialysing at NGO centres	Subsidy of RM 50 if patients fees did not exceed RM 60
2000s	Government subsidy for NGO centre haemodialysis machine purchases	
2006	412 haemodialysis and 31 continuous ambulatory peritoneal dialysis centres nationwide, including at small Ministry of Health district hospitals	

2.4 Background and context

From its very beginning in the late 1960s and early 1970s, dialysis enjoyed the support of influential clinicians and politicians. For instance, on its founding in 1970, the first president of the National Kidney Foundation was the incumbent Health Minister. Members of the Foundation and its Board of Governors have included senior nephrologists, deputy health ministers, politicians, prominent social activists and, since 1996, representatives from the Ministries of Health and Finance.

Among the critical decisions that have contributed to the rapid growth in NGO and private dialysis provision were the following:
1. The series of policy decisions between 1999 and 2001 that increased public financing for dialysis from various sources.
2. The decision to purchase dialysis services from the private and NGO sectors with these increasing public financing, thus instituting a purchaser-provider split. This is a significant departure from the standard integrated public sector approach in Malaysia.
3. Nephrologists' consent to allow non-specialists to operate dialysis centres, staffed at a higher ratio of trained dialysis nurses to nurse's aides, a policy that has only recently been reversed.
4. Provision of a dialysis nurses' training programme that accommodated private sector employees.
5. Minimal regulation: the policy of "treat first, regulate later" where regulation of private dialysis centres has been introduced only recently.

Without liberalization, it is doubtful if the rapid growth in treatment from the 1990s would have been possible. Patients quickly filled up any new capacity created.

Provision of dialysis by all three sectors continued to grow steadily throughout the 1990s. The Asian financial crisis of 1997 failed to dampen this growth. By the end of the 1990s, the Ministry of Health, now freed from meeting urban needs, started to focus the expansion of its services to rural areas that remained excluded. Under a programme of expansion of services, new haemodialysis units were opened in small district hospitals throughout the country so that, by the mid-2000s, every district in Malaysia had at least one Ministry of Health haemodialysis unit.

3. Development of strategy and evidence

3.1 Methodology

Evidence on the horizontal equity of dialysis services was obtained by analyzing data on dialysis treatment from the National Renal Registry, segregated by state (12 political units) and provider sector (three sectors). These data were used in conjunction with state-level population statistics from the Department of Statistics, Malaysia, and state-level household income statistics from the Malaysia Plan reports of the Government[7,8] to calculate the difference in dialysis treatment provision between states and the concentration indices of dialysis treatment in Malaysia overall and by sector for the years 1997 and 2004.

Horizontal equity was illustrated using a concentration curve that plots the cumulative proportion of the population ranked from lowest to highest socio-economic status (income) on the Y axis against the cumulative proportion of health care (dialysis treatment) on the

X axis. Equality in the distribution of health services is represented by a diagonal "line of equality." Concentration curves below the line of equality indicate that health services are concentrated towards the well-off while curves above the line of equality indicate distribution of services that favour the poor: the further away the concentration curve is from the diagonal line of equality, the more unequal the distribution of services.[3]

The concentration index (C) summarizes the extent of inequality into a single index number. C ranges in value from minus one to one and has a value of zero when there is equal distribution of health services. Values of C further from zero indicate greater inequality.

3.2 Evidence

Dialysis provision has expanded rapidly from 1997 to 2004 from 56.3 per million population (pmp) to 119.1. The expansion seems to have been most rapid, however, in the economically advanced states, while the poorer states in the north, on the east coast and in East Malaysia continue to lag behind in treatment availability, as Figure 4 shows. Table 4 shows that states with the lowest treatment rates have seen the greatest *relative* increase but still lag behind higher-rate states by a large amount.

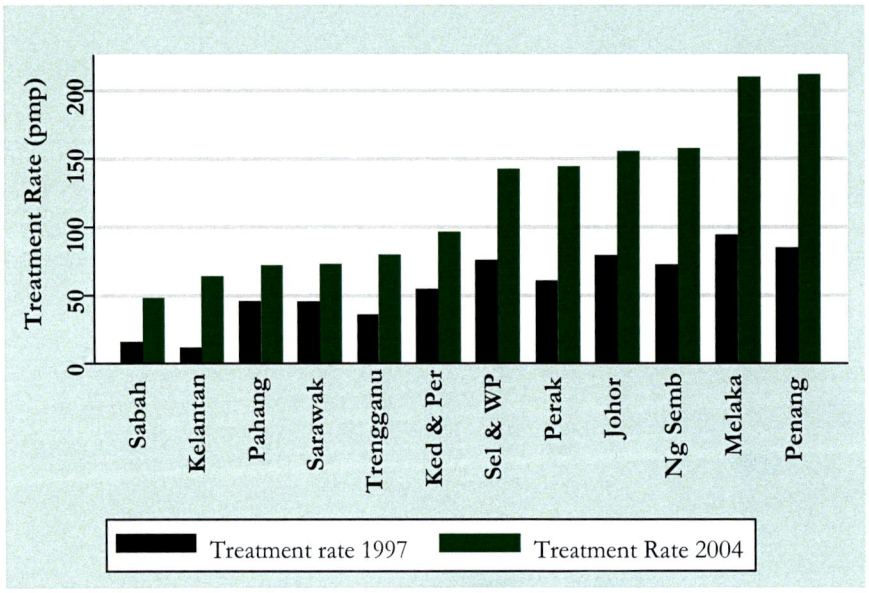

Figure 4: Dialysis treatment by state 1997-2004

Source: Malaysian National Renal Registry. Annual reports of the Malaysian Dialysis and Transplant Registry 2003-2007.[4]

---

3   C equals twice the area between the between the line of equality and the concentration curve. Applied to grouped data (states), C can be calculated by applying the formula suggested by Brown:

$$C = 1 - \sum_{i=0}^{k=1}(Y_{i+1} + Y_i)(X_{i+1} + X_i)$$

where Yi is the cumulative proportion of health services over k groups and X is the cumulative proportion of population ranked by socio-economic status.

Table 4: Dialysis treatment rates, per million population (pmp) 1997-2004

	1997	2004	Change (%)
Malaysia (all)	56.3	119.1	112%
Lowest treatment rate states	**11.8**	**48.3**	**309%**
25th percentile	40.7	72.6	78%
Median	58	119.4	106%
75th percentile	77.8	157	102%
Highest treatment rate states	94.5	212.1	124%
Variation in treatment provision			
Range ratio	8.0	4.4	-45%
Inter-quartile ratio	1.9	2.2	13%
Provision by sector			
Government	54%	35%	-35%
Charitable	27%	31%	15%
Private	19%	34%	81%
Household income (US$/month)	2606	3249	20%
Concentration index			
Malaysia	0.111	0.053	
Government	0.037	-0.047	
Charitable (NGO)	0.294	0.207	
Private	0.376	0.23	
Household income inequality (Gini coefficient)	0.47	0.462	

Sources: Malaysian National Renal Registry. Annual reports of the Malaysian Dialysis and Transplant Registry 2003-2007,[4] Mid-term review of the 7th Malaysia Plan 1999[7], 9th Malaysia Plan 2006.[8]

Figure 5 illustrates the large variations in the provision of renal replacement therapy among Asian countries, ranging from 33 pmp in Pakistan to 1857 pmp in Japan. Figures 1 and 3 suggest that the provision of dialysis in Malaysia and elsewhere in Asia is driven by levels of income and thus affordability.

Figure 5: Renal replacement therapy and income in Asia, 2003-2004

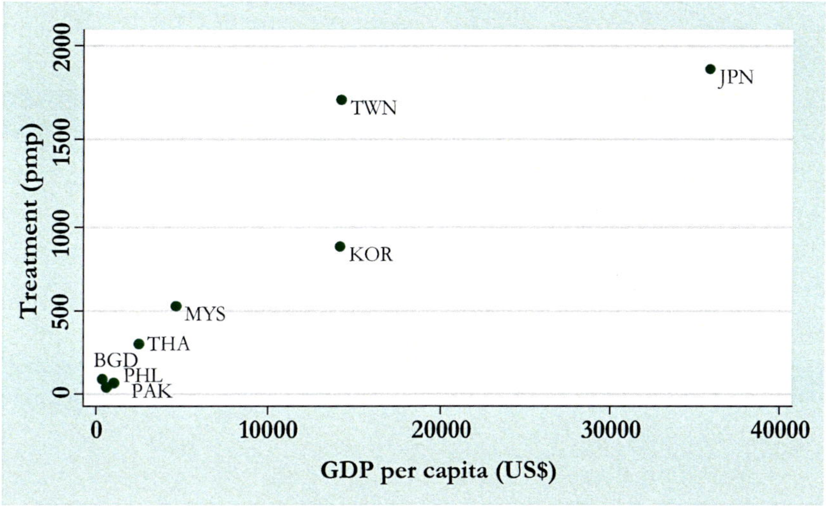

Sources: Malaysian National Renal Registry[11], United States Renal Data System 2006 Annual Data Report.[4]

Figure 6 plots the cumulative population ranked by mean household income (X-axis) of states in Malaysia against cumulative dialysis treatment rates (Y-axis) for 1997 and 2004. The distribution of dialysis is consistently unequally distributed to favour the economically well-off states but, as Table 4 shows, the extent of inequality has declined from 1997 (C=0.111) to 2004 (C=0.053).

This analysis is based on income levels of states rather than of individual patients. The extent to which dialysis services are captured by the well-off cannot be determined directly. However, services in district hospitals tend to serve the poorer rural population and dialysis patients in most public hospitals are over-represented by the poor (see Figure 2).

Figure 6: Concentration Curves of Dialysis, 1997-2004

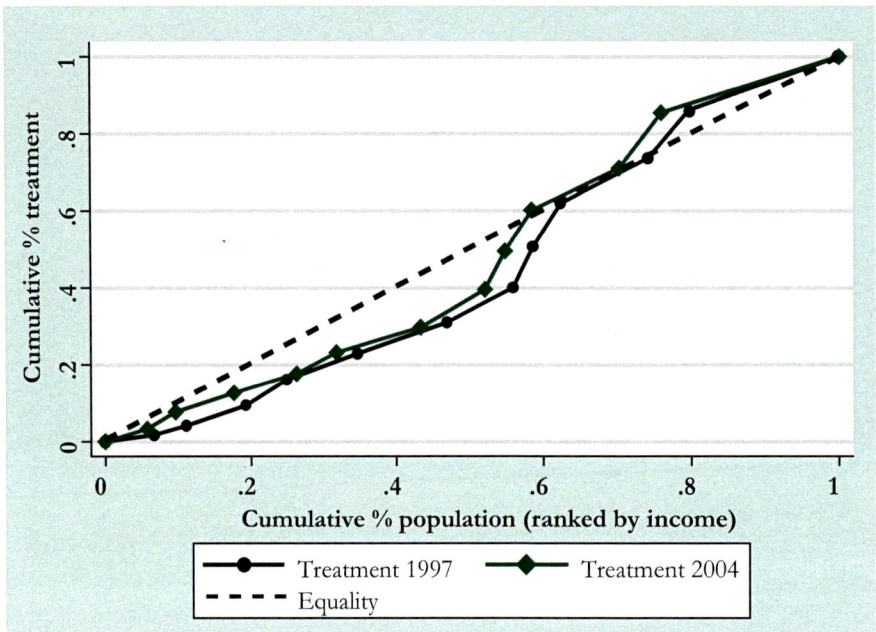

Figures 7.1 and 7.2 plot the concentration curves by sector of dialysis treatment provision in 1997 and 2004 separately and show that government dialysis has gone from marginally favouring the economically advantaged states in 1997 (C=0.037) to favouring the disadvantaged states in 2004 (C= -0.047). Table 4 shows that, although the charitable and private sectors continue to be unequally distributed towards the economically advantaged states, the extent of inequality has declined from 1997 (C=0.294 and 0.376) to 2004 (C=0.207 and 0.23).

3.3 What health outcomes were achieved?

The distribution of dialysis services broadly confirms our expectation that the private sector has concentrated its facilities in economically developed states where patients are able to afford its services, while the public sector behaves in exactly the opposite fashion in accordance with its social equity mission.

The improvement in geographic equity over time might be explained by the fact that the public sector, having been freed from meeting urban needs, could channel its funding at direct supply-side subsidies by locating its dialysis facilities in areas with poorly contestable markets

Figure 7.1: Concentration Curves of Dialysis by Sector, 1997

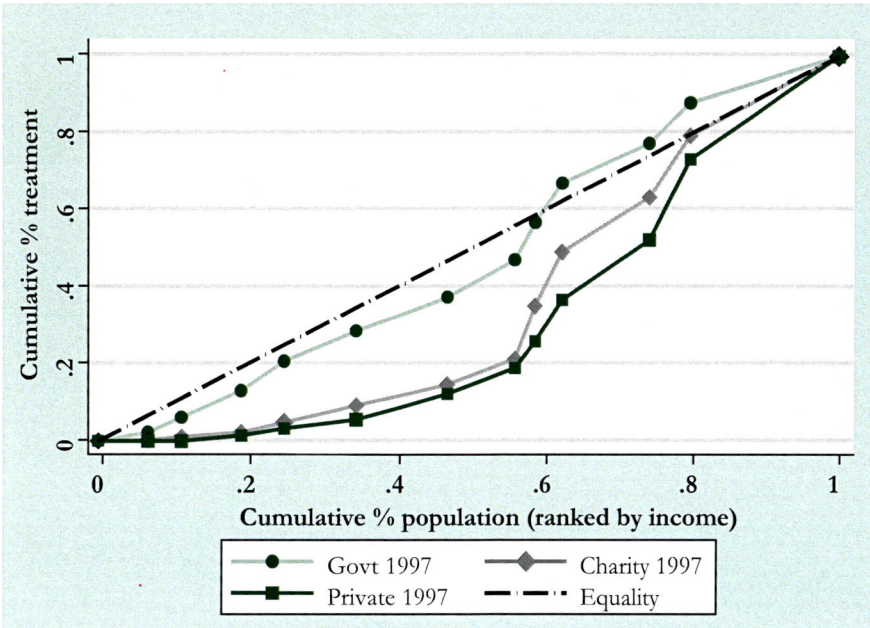

Figure 7.2: Concentration Curves of Dialysis by Sector, 2004

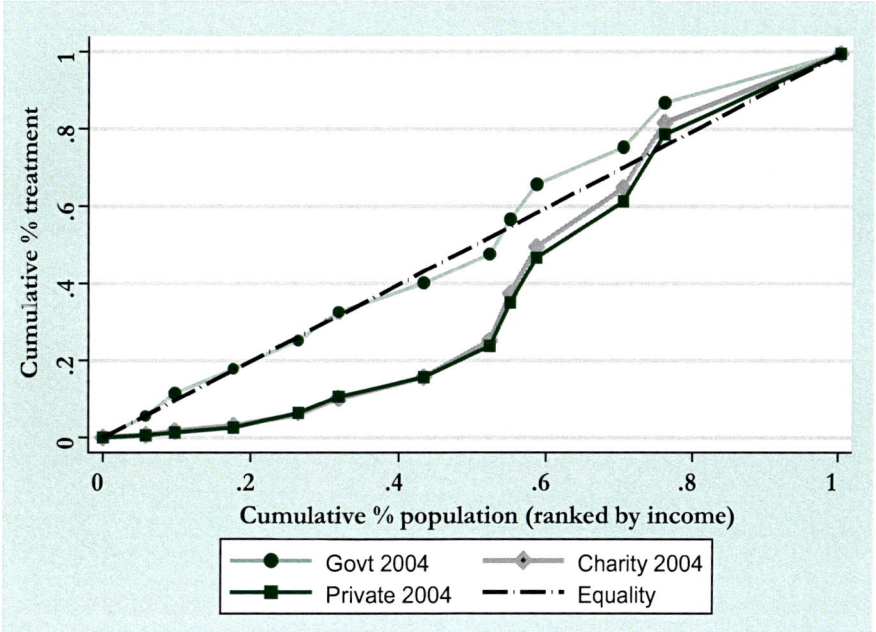

such as rural areas. The share of government sector dialysis has declined (see Figure 3) but the total provision of dialysis has increased across all sectors in absolute terms (see Figure 1). Thus, even if the public share of total provision is decreasing, the number of patients on dialysis at government facilities has increased in absolute terms and is coupled with the targeted expansion of government provision to poorer regions down to the districts. This means that more poor patients from the poorer states are able to access treatment than previously, when services were virtually non-existent or involved long distance travel.

More interestingly, the increasingly dominant private provision of services has not been accompanied by greater inequity, despite the perception that profit-oriented private providers would avoid less affluent areas. Instead its distribution of dialysis services has improved over time too. This might be explained by the fact that the markets for dialysis services in the affluent states are already saturated, thus compelling the private sector to seek opportunities in less affluent locations. We would expect the diffusion of private providers to the peripheral states to continue as incomes in these places continue to rise in line with economic growth throughout the country.

A recent study[13] on the benefit incidence of public sector health spending reports that the Malaysian public health sector has been relatively successful in providing equitable health care, as measured in terms of the targeting of public health subsidies towards the poor. The research also reported that the concentration indices of inpatient care in the public sector were marginally pro-poor (C between 0 and -0.1) while private sector inpatient care was heavily pro-rich (C greater than 0.4). The similarity in inequality estimates between the distribution of dialysis and inpatient care is striking. In both instances, public provision is marginally pro-poor while private provision is pro-rich. This, and the fact that the inequality of dialysis is less than household income inequality in Malaysia (Table 4), as measured by the Gini coefficient, indicates that public sector has managed to play its complementary role in ensuring equity in access to health care.

The only other data we could find to compare Malaysia's experience with is from Mexico, which is also a middle income economy. In Mexico, services are provided by the public sector but operated as separate segments, depending on the insurance status of the population—that is, the insured (comprising employees in the formal sector and government workers) and the uninsured (comprising the self-employed who have no private insurance and those from in the informal sector). A study from the Mexican state of Jalisco[14] reported that, from 1998 to 2000, dialysis treatment rates among the insured population were 5.7 times greater than those among the uninsured (939 pmp against 166 pmp). Only three programmes provided dialysis for the uninsured (as opposed to 15 for the insured). All three were located in the state capital and were thus inaccessible to the rural population, who were more likely to be lacking insurance in the first place. These findings from Malaysia and Mexico contradict the seemingly obvious assertion that public provision is necessary to assure equitable access, and that private provisioning is incompatible with equity objectives.

4. Conclusions and final results

Malaysia's experience as a middle income developing country in providing a costly treatment with scarce available resources shows that:

1. Increase in treatment and the resulting improved access to dialysis is driven by economic development, which translates health care needs into effective demand.
2. Growth in provision has been driven by rapid growth in the NGO and private sectors that, as expected, were highly responsive to market signals.
3. The increase in the availability of treatment and the shift to NGO and private provision has resulted in:

a. improved equity over time and the diffusion of service provision to less profitable areas due to competition, and
b. improved equity of public sector provision.

Endnotes

1. Donaldson, C. and K. Gerard. *Economics of Health Care Financing: The Visible Hand.* MacMillan, 1993.
2. World Health Organization. Equity. Available at: www.who.int/healthsystems/topics/equity/en (accessed 19 January 2009).
3. Hooi L.S. *et al.* Economic evaluation of centre haemodialysis and continuous ambulatory peritoneal dialysis in Ministry of Health hospitals, Malaysia. *Nephrology* (Carlton), 2005, 10(1):25-32.
4. Malaysian National Renal Registry. Annual reports of the Malaysian Dialysis and Transplant Registry. Available at: http://www.msn.org.my/nrr/publications.htm (accessed 19 January 2009).
5. International Monetary Fund. World Economic Outlook Database April 2007. Available at: http://www.imf.org/external/pubs/ft/weo/2007/01/data/index.aspx, accessed 19 January 2009.
6. National Kidney Foundation. History of NKF Malaysia 1970-2006. Available at: http://www.nkf.org.my/01_04history.php (accessed 19 January 2009).
7. Government of Malaysia. *Mid-Term Review of the 7th Malaysia Plan.* 1999:70.
8. Government of Malaysia. *Ninth Malaysia Plan.* 2006:358.
9. Wagstaff A., Paci P., Van Doorslaer E. On the measurement of inequalities in health. *Soc Sci Med.* 1991, 33:545-557.
10. Brown M.C. Using Gini-style indices to evaluate the spatial patterns of health practitioners: theoretical considerations and an application based on Alberta data. *Soc Sci Med.*, 1994, 38(9):1243-56.
11. United States Renal Data System. *International Comparisons in USRDS. 2006 Annual Data Report.* Bethesda, National Institutes of Health, National Institute of Diabetes and Digestive and Kidney Disease, 2006. Available at: http://www.usrds.org/2006/pdf/12_intl_06.pdf (accessed 19 January 2009).
12. van Doorslaer E. *et al.* Income-related inequalities in health: some international comparisons. *J Health Econ.* 1997, 16(1):93-112.
13. van Doorslaer E. Equity in health and health care: lessons from an Asian comparative study. Merck Foundation Lecture. London School of Economics, 16 March 2007. Available at: www.lse.ac.uk/collections/LSEHealth/eventsAndSeminars/MerckLecture2007/MerckLecture2007.ppt (accessed 4 September 2007).
14. Garcia-Garcia G. *et al.* Renal replacement therapy among disadvantaged populations in Mexico: a report from the Jalisco Dialysis and Transplant Registry (REDTJAL). *Kidney Int.* 2005, 97 (Suppl):S58-61.

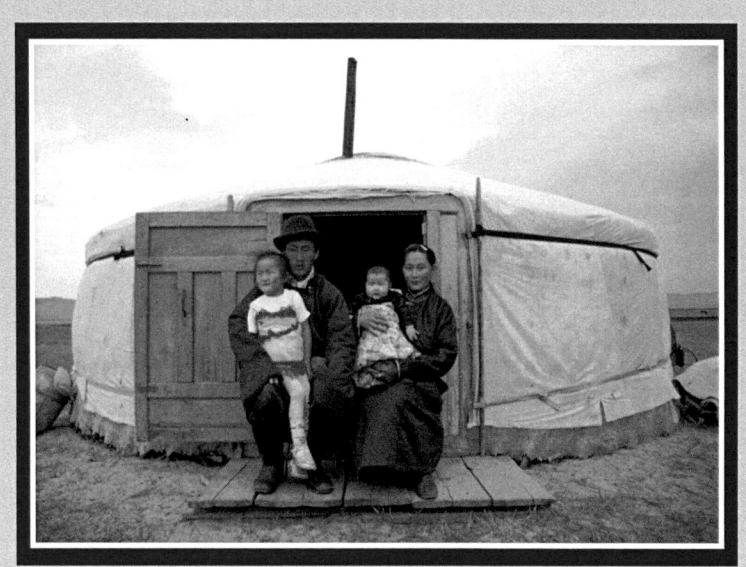

Promoting health equity through capacity building of primary health care workers in Mongolia

D. Amarsaikhan[1], N. Erdenekhuu[2], S. Govind and R. Hagan[3], and E. Nyamsuren[4]

1. Summary

Mongolia is struggling to address human resource issues in its health sector. The uneven distribution of health workers, with increasing shortages in rural areas, is due largely to poor working conditions and a lack of incentives for rural health workers. At the same time, there is an excess of health workers in urban centers, especially doctors. Studies show that income inequality is increasing and inequity in access to health services is a growing problem. Maternal and child mortality rates remain high compared to other developing countries in the region, with marked urban/rural differences. These challenges limit new rural health gains and Mongolia's ability to reach its health-related Millennium Development Goal targets.

For many years, WHO has supported the Ministry of Health in building the capacity of health workers through such training mechanisms as overseas fellowships and study tours, participation of technical and managerial staff in international and regional meetings, and many local training workshops. The fellowships have contributed to strengthening the pool of trained workers. From 2000 to 2006, over 230 Mongolians studied abroad as International Fellows under various WHO programmes. However, despite some notable successes, these overseas training programmes do not always constitute an optimal use of scarce training funds, as detailed in this paper.

An evaluation found that local cost training activities that included district level health workers (and more rarely *soum*-level workers) were uneconomical, due to the very high travel costs incurred by remote participants in coming to the capital city, Ulaanbaatar.

To respond to this finding, the WHO country office allocated some 10% of its regular budget for local fellowships in the 2006-2007 biennium. By the middle of 2007, around 300 remote primary health care workers including nurses, midwives and *bag* feldshers were trained, primarily in the three rural regional medical colleges.

Mongolia has initiated a programme to secure long-term technical assistance to support its human resource development policy and strategies. As noted in its new Strategic Master Plan for the Health Sector, solutions require shared action by many stakeholders, including the Ministry of Education. The Prime Minister now heads a high level committee to address

---

1   Health Sciences University of Mongolia
2   Ministry of Health, Mongolia
3   World Health Organization, Mongolia
4   Darkhan Medical College

continuing issues related to human resources for health. The Government of Mongolia has formally recognized the growing rural/urban inequities and has initiated a range of efforts to reduce them.

WHO has set a target with the Ministry to allocate approximately 15% of all WHO's Mongolia budget in the 2008-2009 biennium for local fellowship training at the three regional medical colleges. Given the wide acceptance of these changes and the satisfaction of primary health workers and their managers, inequity in distribution of health workers between urban and rural areas is likely to be reduced.

2. Purpose

This paper describes an innovative strategy to develop the capacity of rural health workers, thereby helping to reduce the health gaps between the urban and rural populations. Some training resources were shifted from international fellowships to a local fellowship programme. This allowed the training to be better tailored to the needs of mid- and lower-level rural primary health care staff and eliminated several major barriers to the uptake of training opportunities. These barriers included lack of transparency in the selection of candidates, poor English language skills, and the limited ability of many rural health workers to travel and live abroad. Policy changes are suggested based on preliminary evidence that the intervention is effective. It is sustainable and cost-effective, because it costs much less than the previous training strategy and shows signs that it will result in longer retention of health workers in rural areas.

2.1 Background

Several different approaches have been used to build the capacity of health workers in Mongolia. These include pre-service education, overseas training through fellowships, awards and study tours, and in-country workshops and seminars. A large part of donor resources, especially those from WHO, was spent on supporting health worker training abroad through overseas fellowship awards. Evidence collected through assessments of overseas training programmes showed that they had only limited success in achieving the goal of building the capacity of rural health workers. Thus, different options were needed.

2.2 Health gaps between urban and rural areas

Administratively, Mongolia is divided into *aimags* and the capital Ulaanbataar. *Aimags* are further divided into *soums*, and *soums* into *bags*. Presently, there are 21 *aimags*, 340 *soums*, and 1664 *bags*. In 2006, the population was 2.59 million, of which 37% lives in the capital Ulaanbaatar, 24% in *aimag* centres, and the remaining 39% in rural areas.[1]

The health status of Mongolians is improving overall, but gains made in the past through the control of communicable diseases are rapidly eroding, with sexually transmitted infections (including HIV) and tuberculosis, on the rise. In 2006, a total of 36,221 cases of 27 different communicable diseases were reported in Mongolia, which was more than in 2005 by 3,889[5]

---

5 The rate is higher in Ulaanbaatar because all the tertiary hospitals and specialists are located there and all the serious cases from the aimags and soums are referred there for treatment. Thus, the statistics for Ulaanbaatar include these patients from the aimags and soums.

cases. In 2006, the incidence of communicable diseases in three *aimags* and Ulaanbaatar city were higher than the national average. The incidence of viral hepatitis is increasing, especially in rural areas.

Newer noncommunicable conditions, such as heart disease, diabetes, stroke and preventable cancers, are also straining health services, especially for poor and vulnerable populations. Recent surveys have pointed towards increasing trends in common risk factors, such as tobacco smoking, alcohol consumption, lack of physical activity and poor diet.

Overall morbidity is reported to be higher in urban areas, but the incidence of four of the leading causes of morbidity was higher in rural areas. Diseases of the circulatory system, neoplasms and injuries have remained the leading causes of population mortality since 1995 and the number of deaths due to these conditions has been increasing year by year.

In the last 15 years, infant and under-five mortality have steadily decreased. These declines are attributed to the implementation of effective public health measures such as the Expanded Programme on Immunization, the Integrated Management of Childhood Illness and the promotion of breastfeeding. Despite these gains, a wide gap still remains between the urban and rural population in key health status indicators, such as infant and child mortality, maternal mortality, and water and sanitation.

Table 1: Infant and under-five mortality by urban/rural residence, 2006

	Infant		1-4 years old	
	Urban	Rural	Urban	Rural
Respiratory diseases	3.52	13.7	4.45	24.7
Digestive system	1.38	2.98	2.97	5.94
Perinatal pathologies	22.5	28.5	0.0	0.0
Congenital malformations	7.3	4.9	1.48	5.44
Injuries and poisoning	0.6	5.54	13.8	20.8

Source: National Centre for Health Development 2005.

Table 2: Infant and under-five morbidity by urban/rural residence, 2006

	Infant		1-4 years old	
	Urban	Rural	Urban	Rural
Respiratory diseases	19.7	40.7	18.6	40.7
Digestive system	6.19	9.57	5.67	8.97
Perinatal pathologies	4.39	0.8	0	0
Injuries and poisoning	1.26	0.54	4.26	1.33
Infectious and parasitic diseases	0.65	0.37	2.38	2.63
Skin and subcutaneous	1.37	2.15	1.58	2.91
Ear and mastoid	0.7	3.77	0.62	1.94

Source: National Centre for Health Development 2005.

Tables 1 and 2 show data on the leading causes of infant and child mortality, by rural and urban residence. In 2006, average infant and under-five mortality rates per thousand live births were 19.8 and 24.0, respectively. These rates each decreased by one point since 2005, but the rates in rural areas were 20% and 25% higher, respectively, than those in urban areas.

Overall, maternal mortality is on the decline in the country (93.0 per 100 000 live births in 2005), but this is still high compared to other developing countries in our region. The maternal mortality ratio is very high in certain western *aimags*, due to lack of basic essential obstetric services. It is 73.3 per 100,000 live births in urban areas but 105.7 in rural areas. An increasing number of congenital syphilis cases are being detected in newborns at *aimag* hospitals. This is due, in part, to the lack of basic essential services, such as screening for syphilis during pregnancy, in rural areas, and the high costs of going to *aimag* hospitals for these services.

2.3 Human resource issues and challenges in primary health care

Despite making progress in addressing human resource challenges, Mongolia is still struggling to resolve several problems, foremost of which is the maldistribution of health workers. Shortages of key health workers in rural areas have increased in recent years, especially with respect to mid-level workers, who are the heart of rural health care. In *soum* hospitals, one doctor usually supervises the work of 8-12 mid-level workers, so scaling up the training of mid-level workers in primary health care would help improve hospital management and the sharing of doctor's duties.

The quality of health services suffers due to skill-mix imbalances, poor working conditions for health workers, and inadequate facilities and supplies. These problems threaten to undermine the health gains made in Mongolia, with a particular impact on rural populations and vulnerable groups. They also limit the capacity of Mongolia to reach its health-related Millennium Development Goal targets.

The main goal of the health system in Mongolia is to deliver equitable, accessible and quality health care and services for every person. The system is characterized by three levels of services.[5] Appropriate human resource development for the delivery of primary health care is among the significant challenges that the Government and international partners are addressing., Primary care services are mainly provided by family group practice facilities in Ulaanbataar city, and by *soum* and inter-*soum* hospitals in the countryside. In 2006, health facilities in rural areas (*soum* and inter-*soum* hospitals) accounted for 23.2% of the total number of hospital beds[1,6] but served 39% of the population.

Table 3: Health worker distribution in Mongolia, 2005

	Urban/*aimag* center	Rural area
Population	61%	39%
Physician number/10,000 pop.	47.6	17.5
Nurse number	42.3	25.6
Physician/nurse ratio	1.1	0.6
Proportion of health budget	70.6%	29.4%

2.4 Health workforce situation and trends

There were 33,649 health workers in 2005, working in both the public and private sectors.[1,2] Of these, 82% were women, varying from 77% in primary level services to 86% in tertiary level services. While the overall size of the health workforce is considered adequate by international standards, health worker density varies considerably between rural and urban areas. In 2005, *aimags* had an average of 1.7 physicians per thousand population, compared to Ulaanbaatar, which had 4.3 per thousand (Table 3). Half of all *soum* hospitals had only one doctor, and 15 lacked any doctor at all—clear indicators of the critical health worker shortage in rural areas. Geographical inequity in the distribution of mid-level workers is also apparent, although not so pronounced, with 5.3 mid-levels workers available per thousand population in *aimags*, versus 6.3 per thousand in Ulaanbaatar.[5]

The proportion of the health workforce working at the primary or secondary level has fallen by around 8% over the past 5 years (Figure 3). This trend is inconsistent with the Ministry of Health's policy to take a primary health care approach to provision of health services, and to target resources towards the poor and areas in greatest need.[2]

Figure 3. Percentage of health workforce at primary and secondary levels (2001-2005)

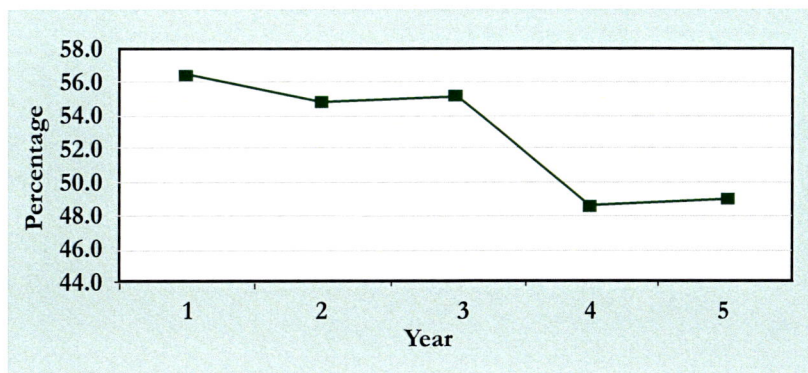

A number of factors contribute to this trend. There are significant difficulties recruiting and retaining skilled health workers in rural areas. The low level of health worker salaries compared to the cost of living, limited incentives for rural postings, and the low number of rural entrants training as health workers, all contribute to this situation.

In addition, poorer socio-economic conditions in rural areas contribute indirectly, by making rural posts less attractive to health workers than urban posts. The high costs faced by rural households in accessing basic social services are one underlying reason for the high rural to urban migration in Mongolia. This phenomenon has been growing and affects all rural professionals. Without good teachers and basic services, mid-level health workers also leave. Maldistribution creates a significantly higher workload for rural doctors than that of their urban counterparts. In 2004, there were an average of 5 doctors per 10,000 population at the *soum* level, compared to 27 per 10,000 population at the national level, and 43 per 10,000 population in Ulaanbaatar.[4] A *soum* or inter*soum* doctor was responsible for an average of 21 outpatients per working day in 2005, compared to an average of eight outpatients per doctor per day in *aimag* hospitals and four in tertiary hospitals. A *soum* or inter*soum* doctor was also responsible for an average of 270 admissions per year, compared to an average of 127 in *aimag* hospitals and 99 in tertiary hospitals.[3] With an average of only 1.6 doctors per *soum* hospital, many rural doctors are on call 24 hours a day, seven days a week, without any other doctor to share the workload.

2.5 Human resource policy and efforts in human resource development

The Ministry of Health's Human Resource Development Policy 2004-2013 sets out human resource development directions and identifies a number of priorities in workforce planning, training, distribution and management. In April 2005, the Government endorsed the Health Sector Strategic Master Plan. The Plan, developed through a collaborative process within and outside the sector, presents a vision for future health services and identifies human resource development within an integrated approach to health services development, as one of the key areas of work for the next 10 years. The three main strategies in human resources for health are:

- to strengthen sector-wide human resource management, based on the Human Resource Development Policy;
- to reform pre-, post- and in-service training for health professionals and workers; and,
- to further develop incentives, including social security, for all health workers.

Many of the complex human resources problems cannot be resolved by the Ministry of Health alone. The Health Sector Strategic Master Plan acknowledges that the process of developing a national health sector human resource development plan must involve partnership with stakeholders from health, education, civil service and finance sectors, as well as professional, donor and consumer bodies.

The Ministry of Health's Human Resource Development Policy 2004–2013 recognizes that the "training of health workers must be closely correlated with ... the health needs of the rural population and the specifics of working in rural areas."[5]

Training strategies to improve staff distribution in rural areas include:
- increasing the quality and availability of training at the *aimag* level rather than requiring students to train in Ulaanbaatar;
- active recruitment of rural students, including through scholarships and contracts, who will return to work in their own communities on graduation; and
- giving priority to rural health workers in in-service, post-basic and post-graduate training.

A large part of WHO's country resources is allocated to supporting the Ministry of Health's Human Resource Development Policy and building the capacity of health workers, through such mechanisms as overseas fellowships and study tours, participation of technical and managerial staff in international and regional meetings and workshops, and local training workshops. This support includes numerous training activities organized for primary level health workers, including clinical, non-clinical and health promotion training for *soum* doctors and bag feldshers, although these have been problematic, as discussed later.

Fellowships offer considerable benefits to individuals and have contributed to strengthening the pool of trained human resources in Mongolia. In 2006, we designed and carried out a study to assess the total impact of WHO-funded scholarships awarded in Mongolia and to provide recommendations to improve the impact of the programme.

2.6 Developing evidence on overseas fellowship training

The overall goal of training is to strengthen the capacity of participants to improve the health of the Mongolian population, with a focus on rural and disadvantaged groups.

The following were the objectives of this study:
1. to assess the success and failures of WHO's current programme of capacity building for health workers;
2. to develop appropriate training programmes for primary health care workers; and,
3. to monitor and evaluate the impact of the programme.

2.7 Methods of the study

The study population included the 89 out of 195 WHO Fellows who had participated in short- and long-term international fellowships and study tours between 2002 and 2006, and who were still in their intended posts.

This study combined quantitative and qualitative methods, including the analysis of routine reports on the completion of fellowships and application of the learning, rapid follow-up studies of fellowships and study tours, and programme evaluations through questionnaires, interviews and focus group discussions with medical professionals. WHO technical staff, Ministry of Health officers, medical professionals, expatriates and other key informants were also interviewed.

The following approaches were used to assess the international fellowships and study tours awarded from 2002 to 2006:
- identifying the Fellows' professional and educational backgrounds;
- assessing the selection procedure for Fellows;
- examining the Fellows' career and professional development upon their return;
- assessing the Fellows' contribution to the health sector upon their return;
- evaluating whether the Fellows' training objectives were met; and
- assessing the limitations and benefits of the Fellowships programme.

2.8 Findings

The Fellows' mean age was 42.9 years,[7] the youngest Fellow being 27 years old and the oldest 45. In terms of their sex distribution, 23 (26.3%) of the Fellows were men, while 66 (73.7%) were women. According to 2006 data, however, 78.7% of the over 7000 medical doctors working in the health sector are women.

There is a distinct bias in the distribution of overseas Fellowship awards by professional category, with 75.4% of Fellows being medical doctors, 5.3% economists, 3.5% pharmacists,

8.8% hygienists, and 1.75% each information technologists, medical equipment engineers, dentists, pharmacists, and nurses. No midwives or paramedics have received awards over the five years.

Nearly all interviewees were unsatisfied with the current selection procedure as well as the information sources about Fellowships. The study found that a systematic selection procedure was generally not followed. The information accessible through the public media about Fellowship programmes for medical professionals is insufficient. The actual practice is quite different from the Fellowship manual rules and procedures, which require that a national selection committee should select the candidates, with the advice of the WHO country office.

Overall, the WHO Fellowships programme still is an important means for strengthening the capacity of human resources for health in Mongolia. The main strengths of the programme include positive impacts on health systems and service delivery. Returned Fellows have contributed to changes in health policies, health legislation and specific disease control programmes. Examples are the new tobacco control legislation, and a national plan for non-communicable diseases control and for cancer control. The IMCI strategy has been successfully implemented in Mongolia with the help of returned Fellows.

In terms of professional development and increased opportunities for career advancement, the Fellowship programme has also facilitated networking among countries and institutions. Mongolia has hosted several international and regional meetings to share experiences on programmes such as traditional medicine, health financing, and IMCI.

In general, however, while returned Fellows are eager to apply the knowledge and competencies obtained from their training, the Ministry of Health has little operational budget to support them in implementing their new knowledge and skills. In addition, neither WHO nor the Government has any follow-up or controls for how the Fellows' skills are applied or what contribution they make to the development of health sector. The study found that, after their training, most Fellows did not return to the jobs they were trained for. Instead, most took up unrelated jobs, for the sake of better salaries or incentives and opportunities for promotion, tending to move to donor-funded projects in the Ministry of Health and elsewhere. This shows that the reputation and value of the Fellows increased, but their post-training assignment experiences are generally not supportive of Mongolia's national health sector development goals.

2.9 Development of Local Fellowships Training Programme

Most health workers in Mongolia, especially those working in rural areas, lack access to international training programmes, mainly due to the language barrier. Since increasing the capacity of mid-level workers would be of great benefit to rural health services, WHO has supported the organization of training courses in Ulaanbataar, but few mid-level health workers have benefited from these short-term (three-to-five-day) local workshops, most of which are related to primary health care[6]. Many primary health care workers have never attended any educational course after graduation from their initial courses.

---

6   WHO supports 18 country programmes covering immunization, communicable diseases, essential medicines, mental health, noncommunicable diseases, health promotion, nutrition, health system policies, and other areas, that involve primary health care workers from rural areas.

Comparatively few rural midwives, doctor assistants, nurses and other primary health care professionals have been trained. A recent survey that included around 500 midwives found that 72% had not had any type of training since their graduation. Not only are they effectively prevented from taking advantage of international training opportunities for reasons of language and selection bias, but nurses and other mid-level health workers are often unable to attend advanced training programmes in Ulaanbataar due to travel costs and distance. Health administrators or their deputies are often the main participants, even though these programmes are intended for technical staff.

Early discussions with the Minister of Health on possible ways to increase the participation of rural or remote health workers were complicated by the perception that Ministry of Health staff and specialists (all urban-based) were more in need of the training offered through WHO's international Fellowships, and WHO Fellowships were needed as an incentive to reward service to the Ministry of Health. In addition, Ministry officials thought that WHO funds should be spent through the Ministry of Health and not through the Ministry of Education. Despite this opposition, discussions were started with the Regional Medical Colleges in 2003 to use their facilities for local training activities.

The objective of the Local Fellowships Training Programme were to upgrade the knowledge and skills of health workers working in remote *soums* by providing accessible, comprehensive training programmes in areas related to primary health care and thereby to improve the quality of health services in rural areas.

Based on the priorities of the National Health Plan 2006-2015, the training needs of primary health care workers were assessed in a process that included:

1. understanding the National Health Plan and the Ministry of Health and international organizations' policy recommendations;
2. analyzing the development of appropriate curricula, teaching and training materials using participatory approach with key institutions; and
3. setting up a national selection committee and transparent processes and sending out open advertisements to inform all health workers about training opportunities.

The Regional Medical Colleges are located in the east, west and central regions of Mongolia. They have long experience in training medical professionals, doctors, mid-level health workers, and nurses. Organizing the local fellowships training programme required strengthening the capacities of these colleges in terms of funds, workforce, and trainers, but this investment has reduced many of the previous barriers to mid-level worker training. It will ensure the long-term sustainability of the locally organized fellowships and the capacity to train many rural health workers. The WHO grant was used to implement training courses in the following areas:[8]

- Pregnancy, birth, post-natal and newborn care
- Noncommunicable disease prevention and control
- Rational use of Mongolian traditional medicine
- Integrated primary health care for rural health teams
- Mental disorders in primary health care

3. Discussion

Preliminary assessment of the Local Fellowships Training Programme shows the following favorable outcomes:

1. Participation of 300 primary health care workers, including nurses, midwives and bag feldshers, have participated in the training and are continuing to work in rural areas.
2. The training has enjoyed wide acceptance and satisfaction among the health care workers, health managers and partners.
3. The Regional Medical Colleges/Health Sciences University of Mongolia and other health agencies have actively participated in the programme.
4. All the Fellows trained returned to their place of work and are supervised by provincial and *soum* level managers.
5. The Fellows have initiated several community-based health programmes.
6. Several additional potential development partners have shown interest in supporting the programme.

The Local Fellowships Training Programme allows training of twenty-five participants at one time, which is a much higher output level than that obtained by international training. It is also highly cost-effective. Between ten and fifteen local Fellows can be trained for the cost of training one international Fellow.

Training modules for each programme were developed with the active and innovative participation of professional partners. However, experience in the two years since it began shows that most health professionals still have a rather academic approach to training. The training programme and modules need to be simplified, made more relevant to the needs of mid-level workers and revised to meet the needs of services at the primary health care level. More active involvement of the Ministry of Health is needed to monitor and assess all training programmes, to ensure that they meet the evolving skill needs of both rural and urban health workers in an equitable manner.

One advantage of the Local Fellowships Training Programmes is that all interested health workers have the opportunity to apply, provided they have at least two years' work experience, a health background, and a willingness to work in their designated *aimag* or *soum* upon completion of the training. Every training course is to be advertised in advance through daily newspapers and websites, and open phone numbers provided for further clarifications.

Feedback has been very positive, with almost all the participants expressing satisfaction with the objectives of the training programmes, quality of training, overall training process, and training materials. Nearly all the rural health workers who attended the local fellowship training faced similar barriers in lacking the financial resources and language skills to attend international Fellowship trainings. In addition, participants support the organization of training programmes in the Regional Medical Colleges because they cannot stay away from their jobs for long durations, due to the rural shortage of health workers. Also, their feedback confirms that this kind of training has become popular, even though it was introduced only two years ago. The Ministry and WHO country office regularly receive requests and questions seeking clarifications from rural health workers about how to apply.

In their feedback, participants requested:

- the organization of more of this kind of training, in every *aimag* if possible, to equalize the distribution of participants and provide an opportunity to share experiences from different *aimags/soums*; and,
- participation by primary care health workers from different disciplines, e.g., midwives or nurses.

4. Policy recommendations

Overall, it was concluded that, to improve the impact of the Local Fellowships Training Programme, WHO and the Ministry of Health should follow a more systematic and diligent selection process and monitor the programme over the short and long term. More specifically:

1. There is a need to strengthen monitoring and evaluation of the programme, in order to improve the transparency, objectivity and effectiveness of the candidate selection and nomination processes, particularly in relation to their job responsibilities, qualifications, experience and language skills.
2. The existing policy aiming to increase the competitiveness and transparency of the selection process needs to be more fully implemented. Mass media should be used to more widely and equitably distribute information on international fellowship training, including through advertisements in daily newspapers, TV and radio.
3. The Ministry of Health should develop a system for ensuring that Fellows apply their newly acquired knowledge and skills by working in appropriate job assignments in the field upon return, possibly through a contract obligating Fellows to work in the same field for two to four years after training. Returning Fellows should conduct a seminar at work to share their new knowledge and skills.
4. Feedback from the participants of the local Fellowship training shows that the introduction of local training was timely and it meets the needs of health workers working in primary health care in rural areas. The growing interest from health workers from all parts of Mongolia also suggests that this training should be expanded and sustained in the long term, based on the capacities of local medical colleges.
5. The training programmes, modules and manuals used for the local Fellowship programmes should have a community health orientation rather than an academic one. These should be revised accordingly and the trainers should receive re-training in the new approaches
6. The Ministry of Health should conduct periodic assessments of both the international and local training programmes to ensure that the training topics (primary health care, noncommunicable diseases, traditional medicine, mental health, etc.) are consistent with the human resource development policy, the overall health sector plans, and the strategy for meeting the Millennium Development Goals in health.

5. Conclusions

Mongolia has initiated a programme to secure long-term technical assistance to support its human resource development policy and strategies. As noted in its new Strategic Master Plan for the Health Sector, solutions require shared action by many stakeholders including the Ministry of Education. The Prime Minister now heads a high-level committee to address continuing issues related to human resources for health. The Government of Mongolia has now formally recognized the growing rural/urban inequity and has endorsed a spectrum of efforts for its reduction.

WHO has set a target with the Ministry to allocate approximately 15% of WHO's Mongolia budget in the 2008-2009 biennium for Local Fellowship training at the three regional medical colleges. Given its wide acceptance and the satisfaction of primary health care workers, and their managers, inequity in distribution of health workers between urban and rural areas will be reduced.

Endnotes

1. National Centre for Health Development. *Health Indicators 2006*. Ulaanbaatar, National Centre for Health Development, 2007.
2. Ministry of Health, Government of Mongolia. *Health Sector Strategic Master Plan 2006-2015*: Mission, Values and Working Principles of the Ministry of Health. Ulaanbaatar, Government of Mongolia, 2005:12.
3. National Centre for Health Development. *Health Indicators 2005*. Ulaanbaatar, National Centre for Health Development, 2005.
4. National Centre for Health Development. *Health Indicators 2004*. Ulaanbaatar, National Centre for Health Development, 2004.
5. Ministry of Health, Government of Mongolia. Policy on Human Resource Development 2004 – 2013. Ulaanbaatar, Government of Mongolia, no date.
6. Mongolian Foundation of Open Society and MPHPA. Report on assessment of master of public health training in Mongolia. 2004.
7. Health Sciences University of Mongolia Public Health School. Preliminary report. Comprehensive analysis of overseas fellowships and study tour awarded by WHO during 2002-2006. Ulaanbaatar, Health Sciences University of Mongolia, 2007.
8. Ministry of Health. Reports and related documents of Local Fellowship training in rural areas. Ulaanbaatar, Government of Mongolia, 2007.